Crownsville State Hospital

Formerly Maryland's Hospital
for the Negro Insane

Meyer Bldg.

Ward # 3

Ward # 6

Store Room

Campanella Bldg.

Patient Cottages

01

02

04

05

11

12

13

16

14

15

MARBURY DR. W.

ROMIG

E. ROMIG DR.

DR.

W. ROMIG DR.

Praise for

MADNESS

"*Madness* is a remarkable feat of reporting, penetrating centuries-old brick walls to reveal in vivid detail long-buried truths about the racism at the heart of our nation's ongoing mental health crisis. Many books are described as urgent. This one actually is."

—Wesley Lowery, Pulitzer Prize–winning journalist and
New York Times bestselling author of *American Whitelash*

"*Madness* is a haunting history of Crownsville Hospital, a segregated asylum in Anne Arundel County, Maryland. Sweeping in its reach, the book—with its use of oral history and a rich archive—offers an astonishing account of the complex relation of race, racism, and mental healthcare in America. But there is something more intimate in these pages: a story about families, about the failures of our country, and about the madness that touches us all. A powerful read!"

—Eddie S. Glaude Jr., Princeton University professor and
New York Times bestselling author of *Begin Again*

"Hylton's in-depth probing investigation of Crownsville's history answers essential questions about what happened to the Black population of mentally ill decades after Emancipation."

—King Davis, PhD, research professor at the University of
Texas at Austin School of Information

MADNESS

MADNESS

Race and Insanity in a Jim Crow Asylum

ANTONIA HYLTON

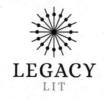

LEGACY
LIT

NEW YORK   BOSTON

Legacy Lit
Hachette Book Group
1290 Avenue of the Americas
New York, NY 10104
LegacyLitBooks.com
Twitter.com/LegacyLitBooks
Instagram.com/LegacyLitBooks

First Edition: January 2024

Legacy Lit is an imprint of Grand Central Publishing. The Legacy Lit name and logo are trademarks of Hachette Book Group, Inc.

The Hachette Speakers Bureau provides a wide range of authors for speaking events. To find out more, go to hachettespeakersbureau.com or email HachetteSpeakers@hbgusa.com.

The publisher is not responsible for websites (or their content) that are not owned by the publisher.

Legacy Lit books may be purchased in bulk for business, educational, or promotional use. For information, please contact your local bookseller or the Hachette Book Group Special Markets Department at special.markets@hbgusa.com.

Library of Congress Cataloging-in-Publication Data
Names: Hylton, Antonia, author.
Title: Madness : race and insanity in a Jim Crow asylum / Antonia Hylton.
Description: First edition. | New York : Legacy Lit, 2024. | Includes
    bibliographical references.
Identifiers: LCCN 2023036585 | ISBN 9781538723692 (hardcover) | ISBN
    9781538723715 (ebook)
Subjects: LCSH: Crownsville State Hospital—History. | Psychiatric
    hospitals—Maryland—Crownsville—History. | African Americans—Mental
    health services—Maryland—Crownsville—History. | African
    Americans—Maryland—Crownsville—Biography. | Mentally ill—Abuse
    of—Maryland—Crownsville—History. | Racism in medicine.
Classification: LCC RC445.M28 H95 2024 | DDC
    362.2/10975255—dc23/eng/20230824
LC record available at https://lccn.loc.gov/2023036585

ISBNs: 9781538723692 (hardcover), 9781538723715 (ebook)

Printed in the United States of America

LSC-C

Printing 1, 2023

To my loved ones.

CONTENTS

Part Four—Black Power and Pathology

Part Five—Where Have All the Patients Gone?

AUTHOR'S NOTE

This book is, at its heart, a celebration of oral history. It is an elevation of the collective memory, experience, and soul of a community in America—a community whose stories have far too often come second. Oral history is as old as any African and diasporic tradition, and a journalist or historian cannot accurately cover our communities without honoring and practicing it. At times, critics worry that the memory is unreliable, that spoken accounts are vulnerable to prejudice and influence. What source isn't? Having spent countless hours reading the meeting minutes, letters, and musings of the state officials who controlled Crownsville Hospital's operations, I can assure you the official, paper record is just as vulnerable to these forces. This book weaves the testimony of more than forty former patients and employees of Crownsville Hospital with the records that have been preserved at the Maryland State Archives and in the homes of former staff members, and with newspaper reports from both mainstream and historic Black-owned publications. These tools complement and do not compete with one another. Together, they breathe life and texture into an institution and an era that has long been misunderstood, whitewashed, and ignored.

This book is also the culmination of ten years of digging through systems that should, in my view, be more accessible to the public in the future. Researchers and interested members of the public cannot simply walk into Maryland State Archives and ask to see Crownsville's records.

They are restricted and carefully guarded, and the state has a responsibility to protect patient privacy. However, as the years pass, I hope more of these documents are made readily available to researchers and to families who might be looking for loved ones and clues.

Back in 2014, I spent months in a college dorm room preparing an Institutional Review Board application and completing training in the ethical conduct of human subjects research and the handling of patient information. To view Crownsville Hospital's records, I would need to be approved by both Harvard researchers and the state of Maryland. I would need letters of recommendation, and have the patience to wait weeks and weeks for someone to respond or process a piece of paperwork. When I would finally get access to materials (and after all that, there were still some boxes I was not allowed to see), I would find that the archives had never received many of the files that would have told me about the patients' lives and experiences. As it turned out, the state had destroyed or lost most of the files preceding the year 1960, and others they had allowed to become contaminated with asbestos. One employee would allege that a collection of files detailing incidents of patient abuse had been shredded shortly after his retirement. So in the end, I had devoted months to studying best practices for handling sensitive patient information, only to find that most of what survived were the thoughts and priorities of those who ran the hospital. I was frustrated, but I pressed on.

Finding patients who were alive and able to speak on the record for this book was incredibly, and understandably, challenging. Most of the former patients have passed on, some are incarcerated, and others were unable to speak with me for personal reasons. Throughout *Madness*, I tried to lift up patient voices through the testimonies, poetry, and artwork they left behind, and through the memories of people who loved them. In some cases, the names and individual characteristics of the patients have been changed to protect their privacy.

I have to thank Sonia King, a minister and former Crownsville patient, whose journey readers will come to know well. When I first cold-called Sonia, I half expected her to hang up. Nobody owes me their story, and certainly not their treatment history. But Sonia was warm, kind, and unafraid. She wanted the world to see how the right mixture of therapy, community, and medication could transform someone's life. She wanted readers struggling with their mental health to know that they are always worthy. That shame could be lifted from their shoulders.

Finally, I spent three of the last ten years interviewing my own family members, too. I felt that I had a responsibility to be honest with my readers about what shaped and motivated me, and that I should do more than just quietly disclose that I come from a family with a history of mental trauma. For several years now, my family has been on a path to change, healing, and discovery. There is no doubt that this experience shaped the questions I asked and the editorial decisions that I made. I wanted to model the kind of self-exploration and judgment-free discussion that I hope my book inspires in others.

American Madness

I HAVE COME TO THIS PARK WITH MY LOVED ONE MANY TIMES BEFORE. Those were good times, when my six siblings, twenty-something cousins, and I had way too much to laugh about. We spent entire days in the park, during the summer and winter, enjoying the gift of each New England season. We tried to teach our cowardly dog to swim in the park's pond and would scoop slimy tadpoles out of the water. It was in this park that I saw a gravestone for the first time, and my father and older sister Ellie explained to me that one day we would all be buried. I didn't take that news well. Still, I gladly returned each time, even as I grew older, to this place that made me feel hopeful. It was a place of family and belonging, where my sisters, my brother, and I would tumble again and again down its little hills and eat the park's snow until we couldn't feel our noses anymore.

Now this same park is a meeting place. It's become neutral territory for familial negotiation. I wonder during each visit: Does every family with a loved one who has been diagnosed with a mental illness have a place like this? A place where two different planets can safely come close without completely crashing together.

Every few weeks in the winter of 2021, I came to this park to walk with my loved one. (They have spoken with me about these experiences but they want to choose if and when they share their name someday.)

They had just returned from being hundreds of miles away. It was the end of the worst year of our lives. My loved one was suffering. They didn't trust a psychiatrist or therapist to get close to them. After calling resource groups and contacts, we were told that there was not a single Black psychiatrist in the state of Massachusetts available to meet with us. The only community mental health service that had offered our family assistance told us that our loved one would be placed on a months-long waiting list for an interview. And when that interview eventually arrived, we were warned that due to the nature of our loved one's challenges, they might miss or misunderstand it. In which case, we might have to start the process all over again.

I was desperate for my loved one to get better, and I was tired of standing in the park shivering. I was starting to despise this place, as it transformed from the soothing foundation of my childhood into a reminder that I had been told I shouldn't go inside my loved one's home any longer. I was also shaking from immense shame. Shame, because days earlier, I had begged a police officer who had entered my loved one's home to tell his fellow officers to never shoot. I had spoken to the officer at a mile a minute, listing every single one of my loved one's credentials. A pitiful feeling had come over me, making me convinced I should try to prove to this officer that my loved one was a good and worthy person.

And I felt more shame, because a not-so-secret part of me was wishing there was a place, an institution of some kind, where I could take my loved one for healing or rest or safety. A place where the experts would be wearing white coats but never gun holsters. A place where doctors would promise me that my loved one was safe, they were sleeping, and they were going to get the best of whatever treatment was available. But because I've studied the history of mental healthcare systems in the United States, I know such a guarantee never really existed. Not for my loved one, anyway.

My loved one believed that they were being hunted by a group of white supremacists. They had covered all of their windows with black gaffer's tape. They had unplugged all of their electronics, convinced they were being watched through every screen and recorded through every button.

My loved one no longer ran the air-conditioning, because they believed this organization had poisoned the air systems with a toxic gas. They were afraid to drive at night. All of their neighbors, from the elderly to the young couples pushing their strollers, had been recruited into this organization, too. Any day now, these neo-Nazis were going to break into their home, my loved one warned. And they would be gone. Please do something, tell someone. Standing in this park, they had not had a full night's sleep in almost a year.

The part that shattered me the most was that my loved one believed I had failed them. They had come to this park to tell me so. That they thought I might have the power to uncover this organization. That I could call someone and tell the story. And in a way, my loved one was right. Every week it seemed there were new reports about extremist and white supremacist groups recruiting members, meeting a former president, joining riots at our nation's capital. My loved one could point to these events as proof. In these conditions, how do you convince the person you love that they are not in the danger that they perceive? The specter of racial violence had become so effective that it was hovering over my loved one without ever having to come knock at the door.

I looked at them, their face now so full of defeat. I had done that, I thought. I felt crushed by the weight of knowing my loved one was about to turn from me and walk out of this park, carrying with them the genuine belief that I had not done all that I could. The belief that I was indifferent to their terror. There was nothing for us to do, no more to say. Everything would keep caving in.

It has been easier to write about mental suffering in my family in a book than to talk about it with friends and colleagues I love and lean on. Yet I feel compelled to write about the history of psychiatry and mental illness due to two forces: fury at the lack of services and support available in this country—particularly for the poor and people of color—and then out of pure, unyielding curiosity, as in both my personal life and in my reporting, I keep confronting this absence of help.

Out on my reporting trips I'm often overwhelmed by how many people I meet who tell me they cannot afford therapy or inpatient treatments that they know they need, that they cannot find providers who look like them or show respect for their personal and cultural experiences. I hear that their sick family members have had more interactions with the criminal justice system than they have with social safety nets or hospitals, and that the more stressors, poverty, and violence they are subjected to, the less empathy they seem to receive from their neighbors.

Social workers, family physicians, and teachers have all reported growing concern about the crisis of mental health in the United States. According to the National Alliance on Mental Illness, an estimated one in five adults and one in six children in our country experience mental illness in a given year. Depression, suicidal ideation, and drug overdose stats have accelerated. At the same time, many mental health services and therapists are not covered by Medicaid and public insurance.

For several years now, physicians and psychiatrists have been warning that the suicide rate among minority youth has been rising. Dr. Tami Benton, the psychiatrist-in-chief at the Children's Hospital of Philadelphia and one of a small circle of Black pediatric psychiatrists, told me that the Black children she serves are under immense stress and uncertainty, and often believe our society is failing to take care of them. On average, they report more than five experiences, big and small, of racial discrimination each day. They face higher barriers when trying to find providers who will take their insurance, and often feel misunderstood by the white doctors who dominate the field. "There's an assumption," she told me, "that when a Black kid comes to the emergency department, the problem is behavioral. It's not depression." In her experience, she has found that less than half of the Black children who come to hospitals and emergency rooms in the midst of a mental health crisis are able to connect to ongoing follow-up treatment.

My loved one says they've experienced the same patterns of condescension and disrespect from emergency rooms to state-of-the-art facilities. All they wanted was for someone to listen to them tell their story and to show them empathy. "Toward the Black patients especially there's an attitude of 'Don't even talk to me,'" they explained. "It's a form of remote incarceration. You're really not trying to deal with the person in a human way." Doctors gave my loved one a diagnosis that was so ambiguous and confusing, it seemed, to them, like "it would have covered about half the population." They left these institutions feeling discarded, and like our whole system was upside down.

In my family, the stories range from regular depression and anxiety to alcoholism and schizophrenia. When I was growing up, nobody spoke about it or made me and my six siblings aware of what resources we might need. We were warned about how much diabetes there was in our family medical history. It would've helped to know about the number of mental breakdowns, too. Still, family reunions and rumors filled in the blanks for us over time.

Without having the tools or the language to talk about it, I became aware of something early: our traumas and illnesses are frequently intertwined with American history and the peculiar reality of being Black. And at times, our traumas would be compounded and exacerbated by poor, discriminatory, or nonexistent treatment when we needed support the most.

Some of the tools and the language came in college. In 2011, I landed on Harvard University's campus as a college freshman, and decided to drop into a lecture called "Madness and Medicine" delivered by Professor Anne Harrington, the head of the small and quirky History of Science department. I got hooked learning about the development of modern psychiatry. I saw for the first time the famous painting of French physician Philippe Pinel casting chains off of "lunatics" at the Salpêtrière Hospital in Paris, ushering in a new era of supposedly humane treatment for the afflicted and a modern, moral psychiatric movement. I read books like Michel Foucault's *Madness and Civilization* and *Birth of the Clinic*, and studied signs of "shell shock" (now known as post-traumatic stress disorder) in soldiers returning home from World War I. I read every version of the *Diagnostic and Statistical Manual* and examined the gendered politics in advertisements for early psychiatric medications aimed at nervous 1950s housewives. I absorbed it all but, frankly, I wanted to know where the Black people were. What has happened to Black people when they, their families, or their communities went mad?

Eventually I stumbled upon a report that mentioned Crownsville, formerly Maryland's Hospital for the Negro Insane. Crownsville was one of the few American segregated asylums with records that had been preserved and a campus that was still standing. Many of the institutions that once served the mentally ill in this country have crumbled, their files destroyed. Some institutions hardly cared to dignify their Black patients' existences with decent recordkeeping. Crownsville still stands, though, and the surviving records tell us a uniquely American story.

What I found was a hospital sitting at the center of a critical juncture in American institutional history—one that Black people played a defining, yet untold, role in building and reshaping. During its peak years in the mid-twentieth century, Crownsville Hospital held about 2,700 subjects, and for decades served as the only mental hospital in the state of Maryland that would accept Black patients. Hundreds of sources—from archival documents, patient testimony, photographs, newspaper articles, government reports, and oral history—paint an image of the asylum as representative of crucial cultural shifts. Cultural shifts in which we needed care but were often neglected, and which ranged from landmarks like emancipation and desegregation to the movement to deinstitutionalize asylums and the rise of mass incarceration.

Crownsville's story runs deeper than one historical hospital in Maryland. It is about honoring generations of patients who were overlooked and mistreated. It's about Black communities and their access to healthcare in the past and the present, and the fight to make space for Black professionals in hospital systems. It's also about the power and potential of having people who look like you take care of you.

As a journalist I'm revisiting Crownsville's story to correct a misunderstood, outdated record. My colleagues often say that as reporters we get on the scene and have the responsibility to write "the first draft of history." And while that's true, I also think our skills and sources can point squarely back at our existing and incomplete histories, and help to complicate them.

My wish is that *Madness* will help us understand both our current, broken mental healthcare system and our carceral one. At the heart of

Crownsville lie a couple of questions: What is the difference between calling a Black patient incurable and deeming a Black population certain of criminal recidivism? To what extent could this legacy be at fault for a current reality in which many communities of color feel alienated by psychiatric services and our prisons and jails are full of people suffering from mental illness? And along the way, I ask doctors, patients, and family what we can do about it.

That day in the park, I did not have the power or the skills to fix things for my loved one. I only hope I have the power to offer something new to you, whether it be greater understanding, an appreciation for our shared history, or just the confidence to share your own family's journey through this country's troubled mental healthcare systems.

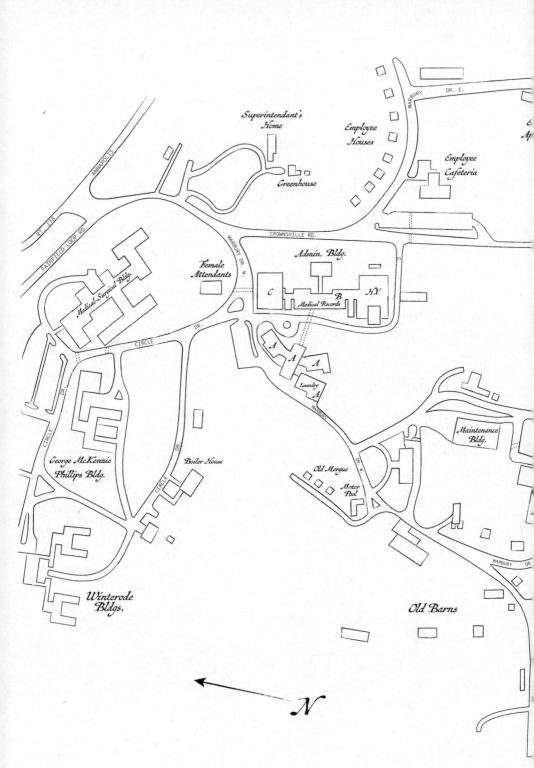

Crownsville State Hospital

Formerly Maryland's Hospital
for the Negro Insane

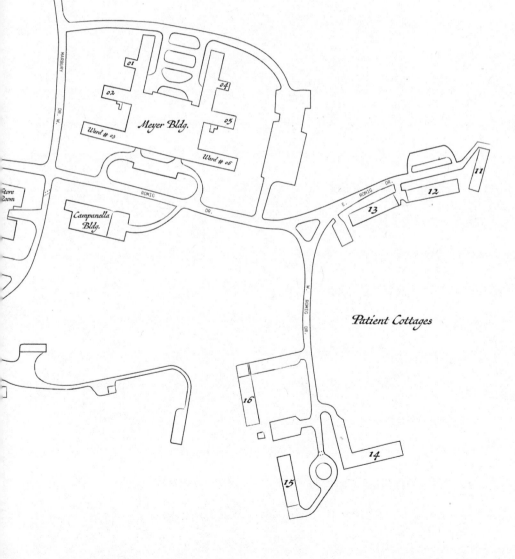

PART ONE

Breaking Ground

1911–1940

1911: **12 Patients**
1940: **1,611 Patients**

CHAPTER 1

A Negro Asylum

Years before William H. Murray arrived at Crownsville Hospital, his friends and six children were desperate for him to find help. By the time he landed on its campus in 1917, his personal and professional life had unraveled. Murray was a graduate of Howard University, a pianist, teacher, and respected school principal. When he walked through Crownsville's doors, he was just another inmate.

The conditions of his segregated confinement at the hospital had been justified by white politicians and doctors as necessary, fueled by a century-long belief that newfound freedom had increased the rates of insanity among Black people. During slavery, the Cotton Kingdom reinforced white dominion and land monopoly; thus, free and enterprising Black communities were a contradiction. Hospitals like Crownsville were one of several solutions for those who seemed unable to survive under the status quo. William Murray was one of the contradictions.

Murray was born in 1872, less than a decade after the chains of chattel slavery were severed, and he had achieved more than many Black people were permitted at the time. But he was having violent mood swings and experiencing depression, which his family believed had been brought on by a battle with typhoid fever and his own stubborn refusal to rest. Typhoid, known as a brain fever, appeared to have changed his personality entirely. Murray transformed from a quick-moving, bubbly guy to an angry, unpredictable, and destabilizing force. Even after a diagnosis, he worked without rest. Out of fear for their stability, his children scattered around to various family members' homes. Murray's behavior caused a strain on his family, forcing them to commit him to the facility.

When he checked into Crownsville's Reception Building, he joined 550 other Black patient-inmates, including men, women, and a small number of children. There were living quarters across four floors and two large hospital wings. Long stretches of time would pass with no eye contact or conversation from the attendants. It could be freezing cold or overwhelmingly hot inside the ward. Photographs taken only a few years before his arrival show men in tattered workmen's overalls, and women sitting in bare day rooms. Many of the patients had no shoes, and in the winter, they were forced to share them. Women wore men's boots. Small kids, living among adults, wore handouts that were too big. The patients lucky enough to have layers were often those working in the fields, sewing in a barn, or cooking in the kitchen.

It was a place where a patient could be locked away in isolation for days, where overwhelmed attendants would, at times, strap wandering patients into heavy oak chairs to restrict their movements, and where people slept in rooms or open porches on thin straw pads. At the time, Crownsville housed every type of patient together—from the criminally insane to those diagnosed with tuberculosis—something that the other, white-only asylums were not doing, and that many clinicians had warned against. During his arrival and amid the First World War, 275 acres of hospital land were under cultivation thanks to unpaid patient labor. Officials were arranging to use patients in their wartime preparedness plans. For weeks, Crownsville's patients would be placed in "emergency squads" and would assist in gathering crops for the businesses and farms in the area for no pay.

The hospital was a world away from the life he had shared with his wife, Agnes, and their kids on Argyle Avenue in Baltimore. There, the family had a backyard where he kept a coop for carrier pigeons and a study where he prepared his students' lessons. He was a teacher dedicated to encouraging academic excellence in Black children, while much of the world around them told them that they were irreparably inferior. But unbeknownst to him and his family, he would never return to that home or that work again after going to Crownsville.

William's daughter, Pauli Murray, would go on to become a celebrated legal scholar and civil rights activist. She would remember his absolute obsession with achievement to be a reflection, or refutation, of the times. In Baltimore, Black men like William weren't expected to be successful. Many were forced to focus on their survival. In the years after Reconstruction, on average, 150 people—almost all Black—were lynched every year in America. By 1892, lynchings peaked at 235. From Tulsa, Oklahoma, to Wilmington, North Carolina, and everywhere in between, a constant drum of racial violence bred a state of paranoia in most Black people, a worry that any step deemed wrong by white neighbors or authorities could end with their body dangling from a tree limb.

Maryland had never joined the Confederacy, although large parts of the state were openly sympathetic to its cause. Still, the state did not outlaw slavery until 1864, a year after the Emancipation Proclamation outlawed the practice across the Confederacy. Throughout the 1850s and 1860s, Maryland lawmakers passed resolutions that barred Black people from assembling for religious events, owning dogs or guns, or being educated, and that limited job opportunities. It was a ban from self-protection, growth, and hope.

By the early twentieth century in Baltimore, it became illegal for a white person to move onto a street that was more than 50 percent Black and illegal for a Black person to move onto a street that was more than 50 percent white. That ordinance was the first of its kind in the nation, cementing apartheid in Baltimore and inspiring other Southern states to follow suit. The ordinance created color lines in Maryland communities that still exist today.

By the time William Murray and his wife Agnes's fourth child, Pauli, was born in 1910, the planning for Crownsville's construction was well underway.

That's also when William started showing signs of severe depression, and his outbursts and mood swings left his wife living in fear. Often

Agnes would flee south to her parents' home in Durham, North Carolina, always eventually returning to him. She was just as focused and ambitious as William. When she and William met, she had moved more than three hundred miles from North Carolina to Maryland, far from her family, to pursue her nursing degree. According to her kids, Agnes was a hands-on mother, the sort who would rush around their kitchen, preparing the family's next meal, all while also sewing and embroidering her next dress. But in March 1914, it all came to a stop when Agnes collapsed on the stairs. William had been on his way out the door, heading to work, when she fell. He turned back, rushed to her, picked her up in his arms, and called for a doctor. But Agnes had suffered a cerebral hemorrhage and was dead within the hour.

She was in the fourth month of her seventh pregnancy. At fifty-one years old, the already-exhausted William Murray had lost his wife and a child. He was suddenly a widower and single parent of six.

Soon after, the Murray children recalled witnessing their dad's increasingly volatile state. He had become more antagonistic toward his children's caretakers, and others in the neighborhood began to take note and taunt them about William's "crazy" tendencies, some even spinning up a theory that Agnes had actually died by suicide.

William's family felt the pressure to send him away. And when they eventually did, they worried about what would happen behind Crownsville's doors.

In June 1923, six years after his arrival at Crownsville, William got into a disagreement with a Polish guard named Walter Swiskowski, who was almost twenty years his junior. As the guard taunted William, he covered his mouth with sticky flypaper. William allegedly peeled the flypaper off his face and returned the favor. As William walked back to the industrial shop where he had been working making textiles that the hospital sold for its own profit, the guard gave a warning. According to reporters at the *Baltimore Afro-American*, he said, "I am going to teach you a lesson." Murray's family was told he said something more chilling: "I'll get that nigger later."

That night, Swiskowski came back. He dragged William to the

hospital basement and bludgeoned him with one of the attendants' bats used for patient management. William was found unconscious and so terribly beaten that he was barely recognizable. He drew his final breaths on a table in the hospital's infirmary. William's official cause of death was listed by the coroner as a "fractured skull from blow maliciously delivered."

The Murray children said goodbye to their only remaining parent.

When twelve-year-old Pauli peered into her father's open casket, she didn't recognize him. His head was purple, and it looked to her like it had been "split open like a melon and sewed together loosely with jagged stitches." The final memory would permanently scar Pauli. In her own words, the stigma of her father's illness and his publicized murder remained the most significant fact of her childhood. Pauli never felt free from the fear that she herself might lose her mind. "This fear hung over my family like a curse," she wrote in her memoir.

William was lowered into the ground at Laurel Cemetery, the first non-faith-based cemetery for Baltimore's Black community. Laid to rest among Union soldiers, businesspeople, and civil rights activists, William had made his way home to peace for the first time in years. Prejudice and racial violence had surrounded him—it had determined where he lived, how he taught his students, and how hard he had to work to advance his family. His downfall, his broken spirit, and his stolen life were the residue of the racial lines that had formed and collapsed around him. It was a bondage to these color lines that even a place designed for rehabilitation could not break. Decades later, Laurel Cemetery would be purchased and turned into a shopping center. William Murray's remains very likely rest under the blacktop of a parking lot.

There was one final meeting before he died: Pauli and her aunt, Pauline, took a train to Crownsville's station. They were nervous to confront William's condition. The station in Crownsville no longer functions today, though you can find old tracks among overgrown weeds when you visit the historic campus. When Aunt Pauline and little Pauli finally made it, they walked along those tracks in town and made their way to the Crownsville visitor waiting room. They watched together as other patients embraced their loved ones. For hours, there was no sign of William.

Finally, in walked William—a shell of the man he once had been. Pauli described her father as an "old man," despite him being in his early fifties. He didn't have the same crisp overalls as the other men but instead wore tattered clothing, which he told her was punishment for an argument he got into earlier in the day. He was so unrecognizable to Pauli that she blurted out loud, "He doesn't look like *my* father." William and Aunt Pauline carried on a brief conversation in which he recounted scuffles with other patients and violent encounters with guards. "I want to get out of here and they tell me I'm ready to go, but there's nobody to have me signed out," William told his sister-in-law and daughter. Moments later, a guard announced the end of visiting hours. Of course, William Murray never would get out.

Swiskowski was convicted of manslaughter and sentenced to ten years in prison for the lethal assault of William H. Murray. His defense attorney, Milton Dashiell, was a prominent segregationist and the very same man who had drafted Baltimore's infamous apartheid ordinance of 1910. The city's second segregation ordinance would be drafted by a man named William L. Marbury. Marbury would later head the board of managers of Crownsville Hospital.

❧

In 1944, a group of Black law students at Howard University were debating how to bring an end to Jim Crow. Pauli Murray, the only woman present, surprised the class at her father's alma mater by betting her professor, Spottswood Robinson, ten dollars that *Plessy v. Ferguson*, the landmark Supreme Court ruling that had deemed segregation constitutional when separate facilities were "equal," would be overturned. A decade later, she won that bet. Rev. Dr. Murray became a lawyer, poet, and Episcopal priest, carrying a commitment to justice that sprang from a childhood with an intimate understanding of the vulnerable Black American condition. Pauli played a critical role in the strategy and planning of civil rights actions and legal arguments in the twentieth century, dismantling many of the separate and unequal systems that had thwarted her parents' dreams one generation before.

As an adult, Pauli Murray came across a sociological study, *Social and Mental Traits of the Negro*, that had been published in 1910, the same fateful and charged year in which she had been born. In it, a white sociologist named Howard W. Odum argued that "the migratory or roving tendency seems to be a natural one to [Black people], perhaps the outcome of an easy-going indolence seeking freedom to indulge itself and seeking to avoid all circumstances which would tend to restrict its freedom." Odum believed that a Black person's desire for autonomy and mobility was the byproduct of a self-indulgent lifestyle, that the Negro had no pride in their ancestry, no ideals, and no lasting adherence to an aspiration of worth. In her memoir, Pauli reflects on how the discovery of the paper helped her see her father's refusal to rest in a new light. Her father had fought against these stereotypes and pseudoscientific beliefs through his personal and professional devotion to excellence.

Crownsville Hospital grew to occupy more than 1,500 acres of Maryland's rolling countryside, and its population was growing. When William was admitted, there were 551 patients. In 1926, the census had grown to 722. By 1936, 1,216 patients occupied the ever-expanding grounds, and it had not yet reached half of its record size.

There are no firsthand accounts recorded by the patients at Crownsville in those early years. In old photographs, they are dressed in the same tattered work overalls that William wore. They are clearing fields, making housewares, and harvesting tobacco as white supervisors or nurses stand over them. The haunting racial lines of the outside world were just as visible in the hospital, with white attendants overseeing Black patients, who had come—or been taken—from somewhere in Maryland.

And each day, more patients were coming in than getting out.

Welcome to Crownsville, Maryland's Hospital for the Negro Insane.

CHAPTER 2

All the Superintendent's Men

THE FIRST TWELVE PATIENTS ARRIVED ON MARCH 13, 1911, BUT they were not welcomed to a hospital ward. They were taken to an open field. These men had been transferred from the otherwise all-white Spring Grove Hospital and taken into the heart of the woods near modern-day Bacon Ridge Park. A man named Dr. Robert Winterode stood before them. He would be their leader, their superintendent. He welcomed them to their new home and shouted directions. Together, they began to harvest willow plant, clear the forest, and begin the back-breaking work of building an asylum.

Maryland's Hospital for the Negro Insane, later renamed Crownsville, took three seasons to build. Dr. Winterode, a well-respected physician who had run the men's ward at Spring Grove, took on the new assignment with every hope of efficiency, and with a fervor that was so palpable that it was remarked on in hospital records and gossiped about by employees who worked at the hospital years after his death. He was on-site day in and day out, watching his workers cut wood and carry bricks, and commanding them every step of the way. He was not the type to delegate.

At the turn of the twentieth century, lawmakers in Maryland were presented with a new and daunting problem: rising insanity among Negroes who were free. In the view of many prominent physicians at the time, the end of slavery had created a kind of aimless vagrant who needed to be concealed and incarcerated in a new form of institution. In Maryland, these patients, who had previously lived in subhuman conditions in poorhouses around the state, were often described as infantile at best, or terrors and criminals at worst. And Maryland was not alone in observing that large numbers of Black Americans seemed to be emotionally or mentally unwell.

For more than a century, white physicians across the South had been writing about their theories on the minds and constitutions of Black people. At first, during the height of chattel slavery, many of them believed enslaved people were completely immune to mental illness thanks to the care of their masters and their time spent in the fields outdoors. But a growing number of escaped and free Black populations altered their hypotheses. Throughout the nineteenth century, one doctor by the name of Dr. Francis Stribling created a set of criteria for the care of Negroes in asylums. Primary to his criteria was that Black and white people were different and must, therefore, be treated separately. He also believed a patient's cure should involve work that was similar to what that person did prior to hospitalization. For Black people, that meant more unpaid physical labor. Stribling was the chair of Virginia's mental health commission and a member of the American Psychiatric Association (APA). His writings influenced psychiatry throughout the nineteenth century, and his senior position influenced the state of Virginia to create the Central Lunatic Asylum for Colored Insane in 1870, decades before Maryland had come to the realization that their state might need to do the same.

In Maryland, and across the country, white doctors, politicians, and local-level leaders became desperate to do something about what they believed were poor, unemployed, and mentally unwell Black populations wandering around, taking up space at almshouses, and allegedly "menacing" innocent children in towns. White physicians and intellectuals had long suspected the Negro race would lose its way shortly after gaining freedom.

In 1851, several decades before Winterode's project began, a

well-known physician by the name of Samuel Cartwright gave this ail-
ment a "professional" term: drapetomania.

Cartwright, a physician and professor at the University of Louisi-
ana, wrote about his pseudoscientific beliefs and observations of African slaves. "Drapetomania," he asserted, was the irrational and unnatural
desire of a slave seeking freedom. If slaves didn't have white people to
take care of them, they would regress. He believed that enslaved people who misbehaved and ran away from their owners would develop
drapetomania, and that slave owners who treated the enslaved with too
much kindness could trigger it. In a circulated paper titled "Report on
the Diseases and Physical Peculiarities of the Negro Race" he described
drapetomania:

> In noticing a disease not heretofore classed among the long list of mala-
> dies that man is subject to, it was necessary to have a new term to express
> it. The cause, in most cases, that induces the negro to run away from ser-
> vice, is as much a disease of the mind as any other species of mental alien-
> ation, and much more curable, as a general rule.

Cartwright described Black people as indolent and miserable. He
saw these symptoms as a medical inevitability: "the natural offspring of
negro liberty—the liberty to be idle, to wallow in filth, and to indulge in
improper food and drinks."

Later in his paper, he criticized northern physicians who had "igno-
rantly" attributed signs of mental illness in Black people to the trauma of
having been enslaved. But he did not let their ideas interfere with his own
hypothesis. The possibility that physical abuse, forced labor, and being
owned by another human might produce mental trauma was not of scien-
tific concern.

Decades later, at the turn of the century in Maryland and elsewhere,
many of these attitudes and worries about "insane" Black people were
still lingering in public discourse.

When Maryland's state assembly decided something must be done,
they made clear that it needed to be done far away from Baltimore City.

Cheap land and the ability to grow crops were important. But Baltimore was also the center of white social and political power in the state. In the years leading up to Winterode's appointment, state leaders wrote incessantly about their worries.

In 1905, when the Maryland State Lunacy Commission released its annual report on mental health facilities, members wrote that "Maryland is too much of a southern State to allow the mixing of white and colored patients... There is no doubt of the fact that insanity is rapidly on the increase in the negro race."

By 1906, a new hospital would become a societal imperative. They wrote, "There can be no doubt of the fact that the progress of the negro from slavery has been attended with a very marked increase of insanity in this race." They reasoned that the rates of insanity would only increase, and the state would need to open a hospital as soon as possible.

So in April 1910, the Hospital for the Negro Insane was created by an act of Maryland's General Assembly. By May of that same year, Robert P. Winterode had received his new post. It was his job to make these problems go away.

The need for mental healthcare was evident, but Maryland's biggest challenge would remain: How do you treat the free and formerly enslaved? How were white people to understand what plagued them?

Africans first arrived in Maryland in the 1600s, and their labor, from tobacco and rice fields to the bottoms of ships in the harbor and into the homes of elites, was a singular force that propelled Maryland's economy and political prominence. By 1755, descendants of Africans, most of whom had been ripped from nations in the interior of the continent, made up about one-third of Maryland's population. In some areas, they were closer to half the population. They were forced to work at breakneck speed in hot, primeval conditions. Maryland's Eastern Shore—the birthplace of Frederick Douglass—was home to breeding farms, where owners forced their slaves to reproduce children for sale across the South.

Throughout the 1800s, a growing fear of slave rebellion inspired owners to become increasingly vicious. By 1860, an estimated eight hundred slaves had escaped bondage in the state. Uprisings and rebellions by enslaved Black people led to backlash, and slavers murdered, shot, whipped, and tortured African Americans.

Free Black people were a direct threat and contradiction to white Marylanders' way of life, and some groups began to advocate for the exile or re-enslavement of free Black people. To be Black in America then was to live in a daily state of degradation, violence, and trauma. For most, treatment and support were nonexistent.

By the early 1900s, something had to be done with all of the people who appeared to be mentally battered and bruised. Officials began to write openly in annual reports about their concerns about the way that Black people were being housed and treated. "The beasts of the field are better cared for than the poor negroes at Montevue," they wrote in reference to a facility in Frederick, Maryland, in 1900. State leaders wanted an urgent solution. And they asked that it be done for less than $100,000 (approximately $3 million today).

The state purchased a plot of land for $19,000 in Crownsville, Maryland. When construction budgets were established, the cost of materials accounted for about $75,000. With only $6,000 remaining, the labor would need to be cheap. Dirt cheap. And the management of such a tight budget is part of what would ultimately make an overseer out of Dr. Winterode.

Patients of all backgrounds were given tasks, asked to clean or make crafts, and promised that work could alleviate mental distress. But what was about to happen in Maryland was unlike anything ever recorded in the country. It would be the first and only asylum in the state, and likely the nation, to force its patients to build their own hospital from the ground up. Black Marylanders would have to earn their access to healthcare through hard labor and a return to the antebellum social order.

"This would lessen the cost of construction and at the same time be a benefit to the patients," officials wrote in the Lunacy Commission Report of 1909.

When state officials approved Crownsville's construction, they began recruiting and transferring patients from facilities that were overrun, understaffed, and looking to be relieved of some of the Black men in their care. After the first twelve, nameless men arrived from Spring Grove, it was only a matter of weeks before new patient-workers joined Winterode's work colony.

They chopped down trees and cleared land for future roads. They carried bricks and wood. They mixed cement and poured concrete.

At night, these men went to sleep in a newly converted willow curing plant near one of the ponds. It had hot water for cooking and a cement pit for bathing. Outhouses, or makeshift toilets, could be found out back. The laborers didn't spend much time there outside of sleep hours. By all accounts, Winterode pushed for a rigorous construction schedule and there was little room for recreation.

Come July of the same year, there was progress, but it was clear more work needed to be done. More patients and workers arrived every week. Few were exempt. There were two disabled men, each having only one arm, who were employed as water boys, and a ten-year-old child tasked with helping to cook and to feed his fellow laborers twice a day.

By September 30, 1911, seventy-three patients had joined his ranks. They came from wards, barns, and almshouses, where Black men were often chained to pipes or kept like farm animals, sleeping together on dirt floors in segregated wings. Hospital records describe them not as patients, but as "charges," whose labor was desperately needed to help Winterode's men use cross ties to extend a spur from the railroad so new materials could reach the property. The men were labeled as "murderers" and "dangerous," as having lived in cells and spent their days in straitjackets. Dr. Winterode was waiting for them. He opened with an onboarding of sorts, letting the men before him know what they were brought here to do.

"He told them that they would be treated entirely differently," wrote a doctor named Hugh Young. "That they would live in the open air and be far healthier and happier. Giving each man an axe and taking one himself, the entire party proceeded to the nearby woods and began cutting the cross ties. The dangerous insane worked with sharp-edged tools all summer and no tragedy occurred."

As the weeks wore on, the acreage expanded. Where there was once a thick forest, there were now the early signs of a fertile farm. Patient-laborers arrived from new corners of the state. More men made the same journey on a ride to the local terminal station or in cars on winding country roads to the work camp in the middle of nowhere. After they finished construction on the main buildings, women would join them, too.

The laborers pushed wheelbarrows of concrete up steep hills, assisted electricians and plumbers with infrastructure, and maintained the sleeping spaces and laundry of those working on-site. Some excavated the land for the foundations of buildings. Other laborers tended to the food: corn, cabbages, tomatoes, radishes, onions, peas, beans, potatoes, watermelon, and cantaloupes. There was a never-ending list of work to be done and no shortage of carriers to do it. Soon the completed layout would include four cottages arranged in a quadrangle, an administrative building, a central kitchen, and a communal dining space.

Near the end of construction in March 1912, a fire broke out, forcing Winterode's men to flee and find shelter in barns a mile and a half away

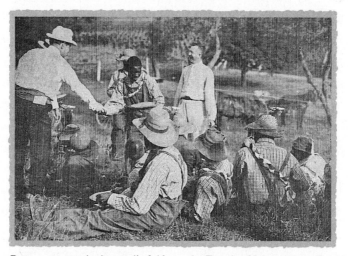

Patients rest in the hospital's fields on the Fourth of July in 1912. From the collections of the Maryland State Archives.

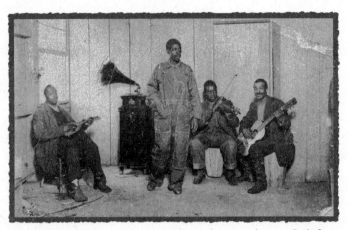

A group of patients play music together in between their work shifts in January of 1913. From the collections of the Maryland State Archives.

from the future campus. For about two weeks, the project ground to a halt. But he made sure to not lose much ground. The patients were sent to live in shacks as they continued construction, and Winterode came to stay with them. He was always near them, always monitoring. He even had a telephone installed and hung from a cherry tree outside of the makeshift shacks where he and his workers toiled.

Within two weeks, his budding farm colony had repaired the fire-damaged dormitories. He brought in sixty more patients to finish the job.

By October 1912, almost 150 patient-laborers were living on-site. Around this time, patients were beginning to be brought in by law enforcement. "It is the exception if patients are brought by any other than the deputy sheriff," read one Lunacy Commission report from December 1913. "Who knows absolutely nothing of them or their relatives, having seen them just a few hours after leaving the jail."

Once construction was complete, Winterode was proud of what he had helped birth: Crownsville Hospital was standing tall, the product of its future patients. A place that conveniently became both a solution to white Marylanders' concerns and a pen for the Black people who'd just built it.

The hospital would employ Winterode as superintendent for more than three decades, and he'd continue to lead every aspect of Crownsville's daily operations with an iron fist.

The campus became the home for Black people who were mentally unwell, "feebleminded," maladjusted. Or, in many cases, simply unwanted. They would come, or be brought, to Crownsville to be healed and rehabilitated. For decades, they would be more likely to die there than find their way home.

The laborers who had toiled over the grounds were marched inside the buildings, into rooms they had hammered into place, and admitted as the very first patients. But that would not mark the end of their days of work. In addition to planting and harvesting crops on the Crownsville campus, the patients "were taken in motor trucks to adjoining farms within a radius of ten miles," where they "gathered the crops for the farmers who were without help." The twenty-eighth Lunacy Commission report boasted about how useful it was to have a captive work force that they could send about town. "This is only a demonstration of how practical it is to have a group of patients under the supervision of a careful attendant."

Crownsville's origin established patterns that would haunt the asylum for its ninety-three years in operation. Early records and photos of Crownsville's founding led me to question America's legacy of race in mental health: What does it mean to be healthy and well enough to clear the woods, build a road, and construct a hospital, yet also be so sick you require institutionalization? How do we decide who's irredeemable and who's capable of recovery? What role have men like Robert Winterode played in alienating Black patients from therapy and care?

Crownsville positioned itself as the answer to "Negro insanity," with little interest—at least as reflected in the public record—in exploring why Black people were suffering in the first place. Crownsville sought to unburden the rest of the state of Maryland from a Black population who appeared unable to adjust to the way things were and whom leaders wanted out of the public eye. And if the plan could be carried out in a cost-effective way in the eyes of the Maryland legislature—even better.

By 1920, the Crownsville Hospital property was worth almost half a million dollars. There to serve the more than five hundred patients at the time were two physicians and seventeen nurses. That year, twenty-eight patients were discharged as improved, eleven more were sent home despite a lack of improvement, and a shocking ninety-seven people died.

What started as a three-building structure built by patients grew to a massive operation, home to thousands of patients, thousands of employees, dozens of buildings, sheds, and cottages, hundreds of acres of farmland worked by patients, and a large mansion for superintendents to live in.

The Crownsville campus, with its mix of residential and recreational spaces for patients and employees, became a microcosm of the state of Maryland. Ultimately, the history of Crownsville provides a window into the past and future of mental healthcare for Black Americans. Who cared for the Black people behind the walls? And who cares to now?

CHAPTER 3

The Sea, the Farm, and the Forest

T HEY CAUGHT THEIR FIRST GLIMPSE OF THE CHESAPEAKE FROM cargo ships. Aboard these monstrous, rancid vessels, they saw a shoreline that glistened blue green at the surface and sparkled where the water met the warmth of a foreign orange sun. The enslaved Africans brought into the Severn River would have seen sails flapping on old ketches, and small dugouts swinging on the shore. They could hear the racket of the dock—the sounds of drunken sailors, businessmen, and auctioneers, all anticipating their arrival.

The history of Annapolis and Anne Arundel County, and the place of their Black citizens, is told out on the water. It was a beginning and an end all in one. The slave ships would creep in toward the docks but never get too close to shore. Historians believe this may have helped prevent escapes. Others grew up hearing that the stench from slave ships was too much for white Annapolitans to bear, and so they were asked to keep some distance.

There was no auction block in the town square. Enslaved people were instead sold off in private, in nearby bars, or sold into slavery directly from the ship, before their feet had ever touched American soil. In some cases, prominent white families would personally finance dozens of these voyages and the forced enslavement of thousands of Black people.

Today the city of Annapolis seems quaint and charming on the

surface, and in the mind of many Americans it lives in Baltimore's boisterous shadow. But the city is not just Maryland's capital—it was once
our nation's. The Treaty of Paris was ratified here in January 1784, marking an official end to the Revolutionary War. It is also the site where on
September 29, 1767, Kunta Kinte allegedly arrived in America aboard a
ship called *Lord Ligonier* and was sold into bondage by a man named John
Ridout. Author Alex Haley told the infamous, semi-fictionalized account
of his ancestor in *Roots*, and while millions of people around the world
have come to know his heritage, they do not always remember that the
city of Annapolis is where Kinte's journey in America supposedly began.

So much of Black Annapolitans' existence was negotiated in the water.
In the summer of 1863, months after President Abraham Lincoln signed
the Emancipation Proclamation, Union troops led by the abolitionist
Colonel William Birney organized a regiment of U.S. Colored Troops in
Maryland. His first regiment was composed of free Blacks who had been
forced to labor on fortifications surrounding Baltimore, and of formerly
enslaved people who had been held in slave jails near the harbor. He
recruited free Blacks and fugitive slaves into his ranks, and with them,
he conducted raids to lure slaves from Maryland's intractable plantations.
They would glide on steamers down the Chesapeake Bay from Baltimore,
and turn into one of several rivers. At night, enslaved people would abandon their masters and join them aboard. They nicknamed one of the ships
the "Jesus" boat. Its real name was *Paradise*, and Birney and Union scouts
promised enslaved people that the boat would transport them there.

According to historian John R. Wennersten, during Colonel Birney's
visit to the town of Snow Hill in Worcester County, a brass band made
up of Black musicians played stirring martial music on board *Paradise*,
while U.S. Colored Troops with fixed bayonets marched through the
streets. This display of force and unity was a powerful symbol of hope,
inspiring slaves and free Blacks alike to flock to the boat and make a
break for freedom.

The mere mention of emancipation sent shivers down the spines of
some of Maryland's leaders. According to Wennersten, they were petri-
fied by the potential loss of over half a billion dollars in property, and the

looming threat of Black political equality. These concerns were especially acute in Annapolis, where African Americans constituted a third of the population in the nineteenth century. Prior to the Civil War, Maryland had more free African American citizens than any other state—some even came to own property. Prominent politicians and slave owners like Congressman John W. Crisfield believed Black people would not be able to handle freedom, that the state was facing a choice, in Crisfield's words, "between slavery on the one hand, and degradation, poverty, suffering, and ultimate extinction on the other."

Black Annapolitans live with a deep awareness that their relationship to the water goes far beyond their work as watermen, dredging oysters, or enjoying summers spent crabbing in rivers. The water is a border and a portal. It is past and present. It's a tragedy but also a passage to freedom.

Today many of the city's Black residents describe a community in which Black and white people share public space but remain physically and psychologically separated. Everything from the water to the architecture to the local cemeteries carries different meanings for them. Many of the prominent white families that still live in the area were slave owners, and many of the historic Black families carry the surnames of their former oppressors, having long been cut off from their own heritage.

Janice Hayes-Williams, a local historian and community organizer, is one of them. Her ancestors sailed the Chesapeake and landed in Annapolis before America was a country. She's tall, with high cheekbones and piercing eyes, but unlike most researchers and history buffs, she's typically found wearing a pair of Timberland boots and rarely seen inside an office. When Janice goes out into Annapolis to hold events and give professional tours, she's known to be blunter than most about what happened in her city and at the docks.

Crownsville is a part of Janice's DNA, too. Her uncle, George Phelps, was the first Black sheriff's deputy in the county and would sometimes escort people to the hospital. She remembers growing up sensing that Crownsville's name carried weight; there was not a Black parent in the county who didn't use it as a threat. If you broke the rules, that was where the elders warned you would end up. If you got caught loitering late at night, the rumor was that a "Night Doctor" would scoop you up and drop you off at Crownsville, and you might never be seen again.

As a young adult, Janice didn't understand why her grandmother, Louisa Hebron Phelps, would walk to the bus stop and ride to the hospital's campus to spend days comforting adolescent patients she didn't know. Louisa had been born in 1897, the first generation in her family completely removed from slavery. Janice grew up with her in a humble home on South Street, downtown in a tight, watchful Black community. The kind of place where if you were somewhere you were not supposed to be, someone's mother or grandmother would tell on you. From her grandmother, Janice inherited a spirit of curiosity and the tradition and practice of oral history. But her grandmother had debilitating arthritis, and Janice worried the trips to Crownsville were too much work for someone in so much pain.

It wasn't until 2003 that Janice realized the significance of her grandmother's visits to the hospital, and that she would choose to follow in her footsteps to bring comfort to patients who had no one else in their corner. Out of curiosity, she began traveling back and forth to the Maryland State Archives with a group of friends and volunteers to review every death record from Crownsville Hospital. She wanted to match the name of every patient who died with their final resting place. The first person buried there had died in 1912, in the months surrounding Superintendent Winterode's grueling construction project.

Janice started to call around to friends, reporters, and politicians and let them know what she discovered—some had been buried in local cemeteries, others were shipped as cadavers and used for medical research, and hundreds, maybe thousands, of people had been interred in the campus cemetery without a proper trace. The cemetery of another, historically white hospital called Eastern Shore had already been turned into a golf course. She refused to leave her people behind. She spent the next two decades trying to bring them recognition and dignity.

"When I look for my people, I look for where they are buried," Janice once told me. One of the stops on Janice's historical tour is an old cemetery in the heart of Annapolis. Named after Circuit Judge Nicholas Brewer, Brewer Hill Cemetery is the final resting place for thousands of Black people, including some Crownsville patients, who lived and died in Annapolis. The grass is wild and patchy on its side of West Street. Many of the headstones bend down toward the dirt or are crumbling completely. Many buried there were formerly enslaved by Brewer and his family, including Janice's maternal ancestors.

While the military cemetery next door is pristine and maintained by the federal government, Brewer Hill Cemetery has long depended on the benevolence of local Black families and individuals like George Phelps, Janice's uncle. Uncle George, as Janice lovingly calls him, led efforts to raise about $95,000 for the preservation and beautification of the cemetery. Thanks to him, visitors now enter past a low, solid brick wall bearing the words "Brewer Hill Cemetery." But caring for the cemetery has been a constant financial and communal struggle. For many Black residents, its physical deterioration represents the constant, exhausting fight to be seen and heard in Annapolis. It can feel as though the rest of their city is content to have them buried quietly and overgrown by weeds, whether it be downtown or in a quiet corner of an old mental hospital.

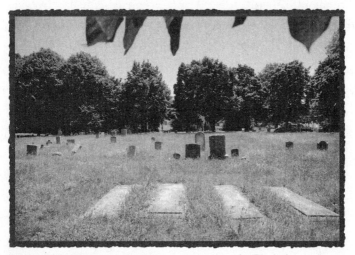

Brewer Hill Cemetery is the oldest resting place for Black Annapolitans. Black families continue to fight for its restoration. But if you peer through the trees, you can see a pristine military cemetery maintained by the government. Photo by Cassandra Giraldo.

North of Brewer Hill, across the Severn River, is Whitehall Manor, which attracts families from near and far for weddings on its picturesque grounds. Its website boasts bright photographs, smiling faces, and a Georgian mansion with the line, "Premier Waterfront Wedding Venue." But behind the fairy tale is a darker story that is not so neatly packaged into party planning. Whitehall Manor was once the home of Horatio Sharpe, the British colonial governor of Maryland, and his many enslaved people. Sharpe, who arrived in America in 1753, held the governorship for sixteen years and kept a sprawling operation that relied on enslaved Black people and indentured white servants, many of whom maintained his beloved gardens. He was a friend and employer to John Ridout, the auctioneer who sold off Kunta Kinte. As it happens, Sharpe was the owner of the paternal side of Janice's family. Once I understood this, I understood why Janice is always joking that she is of the Black aristocracy in Maryland—and why she refuses to let anyone in town forget it.

A few years ago, Janice had a medical emergency. At one point, everyone around her worried that the fiery historian and keeper of Black Annapolis culture would never be the same. Janice, ever the joker, suspected some of her critics were praying on it. And for two years, she could barely speak. She spent almost all of her time hiding out at home and resting with her two adult children, firing off emails when she really had something to say.

One day she woke up in a hospital. Her grandson had come to visit her and was seated by her side reading from children's books, praying Janice would respond. Moments later, a nurse walked in. Janice sat up and blurted out, "What the fuck is happening?"

And from that moment on, her speech started to improve. It was like her brain had taken a few years' rest and one morning reloaded and reset. "I think God wanted me to rest because certain things were coming and my voice needed to be heard."

In the spring of 2022, she and a team of volunteers were on the brink of finalizing more than 1,700 names of patients who had been buried in Crownsville's old patient cemetery.

The vast majority of the patients had been laid to rest without a proper headstone; often there was just a number and no name on a small stone or concrete shaft. Janice helped county leaders secure more than $30 million in funding from state lawmakers to not only order a stone memorial to the buried, but to turn Crownsville Hospital's land into a memorial, park, and museum.

That spring I spent an evening with Janice and a group of friends and researchers, and we plucked rose petals together in one of the hospital's old administration rooms. The next morning, she planned to host a ceremony to honor those who had died and been buried on Crownsville's grounds.

It was time to make Annapolis remember.

On December 27, 1912, Maryland's premier newspaper, the *Baltimore Sun*, published an article announcing that in about a week, the new State Hospital for the Negro Insane would be ready to open its doors to up to 250 patients. In anticipation of the hospital's expansion, they wanted to give their readers a window into its operations and paint a picture of patients' daily lives. The journalist remarked on how unusual it was that all of the work done on the hospital grounds had been performed by patients—"insane Negroes"—who had dug foundations, mixed their own cement, and carried bricks from one building to the next. The *Sun* praised the labor, claiming it saved the state thousands of dollars and was the best known treatment for most mental diseases. The author claimed he spent time with one patient, a twelve-year-old "idiot" (a term commonly used at the time for people with developmental differences) who could not talk and was barely able to care for himself. The article didn't include much more about the child's life or condition. The only detail known for certain was that the patient could not speak. But, rest assured, the reporter insisted, "his hours of labor are now his happiest."

The article introduced two male patients who had allegedly struck up some sort of alliance, calling themselves King Philip and Black Prince. They had styled themselves the leaders of patient life on the wards and had a grand plan to establish their own kingdom. The journalist found their names and delusions of nobility all very funny. The hospital staff put Black Prince to work mixing concrete for the hospital's foundations. But they humored King Philip, an avid reader of the Bible, by granting him control over the dormitories and allowing him to tell other patients what to do.

It was a bleak and unsettling picture. At no point did the journalist pause to consider why these two Black men in 1912 might have been searching for some sense of status and order in the world. The reader is in on the joke. We know who is really in charge on the farm.

Crownsville's self-contained community was isolated from the rural town surrounding it. Few knew what was happening behind this new institution's walls except those living and working on the inside, and small grand juries who periodically toured the state's mental hospitals. The hospital grounds were bisected by a single tar country road, a stark symbol of what divided the staff from the patients and their treatment. The land had once been a fertile expanse of corn and wild grass, but now it was dotted with more than a dozen structures across its 1,500 acres. In those early decades, life was uneventful in this part of Anne Arundel. Passersby could glimpse cattle grazing or male patients working through the day, picking tobacco plants or shoveling coal into the heating plant. In their first year of operation, patients had excavated the buildings' foundations, filled an adjoining ravine, and unloaded hundreds of carloads of bricks, sand, and gravel. Despite its bucolic appearance, Crownsville was a modern, highly productive farm—one that was able to produce much of its own food and even practice irrigation, all thanks to the labor of its patients. But that idyllic facade helped to mask a darker truth behind its walls.

Being institutionalized at Crownsville was like serving a sentence. Time didn't stand still so much as it simply did not matter. Because Crownsville served as the sole psychiatric institution catering to Black patients from across the state, some patients found themselves cut off from the outside world and many miles from relatives living in far corners of Maryland. With family ties often frayed or nonexistent, many of those

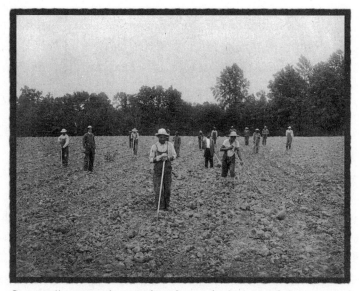

Crownsville patients harvested produce and tobacco, tended to cows and horses, and served meals to their fellow patients and the staff. From the collections of the Maryland State Archives.

under its care had few visitors. The demands of daily life often meant that relatives simply lacked the time or resources to make the long journey to Crownsville. This isolation only served to compound the pain of those struggling with mental illness, rendering them even more invisible—and bound to their endless list of day-to-day chores.

There was a receiving ward made of three interconnected structures— at the center stood an infirmary flanked by two dormitories. Dozens of the patients lived out in wood-frame shacks.

When it was mealtime, patients would drop the sticks and tobacco spears that they used for work and file in from the fields. Older and able-bodied patients would help bring meals to the youngest and those with disabilities, like they were their own kin. If a patient had been seated inside all day, it was a sign that staff believed they couldn't help keep this place running.

Constant patient labor had two benefits: first, according to physicians like Samuel Cartwright and the leadership of Maryland's Lunacy Commission, it was the key to these patients' recovery, and second, it was a convenient way to keep hospital costs down. The female patients often toiled away washing and mending clothes and repairing shoes. Whether doing laundry, weaving baskets, cooking, or transporting other patients, Crownsville patients were constantly offsetting the costs of their own care.

And when they were done cleaning up after themselves, they took care of the staff, too. A select group of trusted patients would be tasked with serving Superintendent Winterode and his top lieutenants each of their meals in a private dining room. They would then carry trays of food out to the rest of the staff, like waiters working at a private club.

One local report from 1912 described how "the laundry work for the patients is done by two adult males and an epileptic imbecile 10 years of age who has been taught to feed the [w]ringer and at which he has become quite adept. During the past year these three have washed and ironed over 40,000 pieces." Hospital leadership wanted to prove that the hospital was self-sufficient and cheap, and there was an obsessive focus on the work the patients provided in hospital and newspaper reports for decades.

Decades later, in January 1949, a series of local newspaper articles described a Black physician named Dr. J.E.T. Camper, who alleged that patients who were well enough to be released were being held at Crownsville because of the value of their services to the institution. At a meeting of the Mental Hygiene Society of Maryland—an organization of leading psychiatrists and physicians—Dr. Camper stated that he had been instrumental in obtaining the release of patients unfairly held at the hospital and that he believed other patients who could be dismissed were held "in a sort of peonage." Dr. Camper offered his colleagues names, dates, and parental contact information for the patients he had discovered. One was a girl kept as a servant in Superintendent Winterode's home. The other, who had previously been kept at Crownsville as a cook, was now an employee of the Post Office. "The hospital authorities [had been] claiming they needed him," Dr. Camper told the room. "And that keeping him there would 'do him no harm.'"

Patient stays were extended to meet production needs. Patients at Crownsville were trapped in a cycle of free labor—one that began as a questionable form of therapy and frequently ended either in their exploitation by local companies seeking a cheap labor source, or in their peonage and service to the very hospital and state that was intended to earnestly facilitate their rehabilitation.

Patient labor was big business for Crownsville, both on-site and off. Employees recognized this dynamic for what it was—a direct outgrowth of the labor and racial hierarchy that had existed in Maryland for their entire lives. I spoke with three former employees who grew up in Annapolis and Baltimore and recalled that well into the 1960s, it was common knowledge that Crownsville patients were rented out to local companies looking for cheap labor. Two of the employees were told that the patients were paid about fifty cents per day. While they might receive a part of their wages, most would go to offset the cost of their care at the hospital. During the early 1940s, as white Marylanders left to fight in World War II, Black patients at Crownsville were recruited to fill vacancies on local farms. One former employee remembered seeing local companies post bigoted signs down West Street in Annapolis, and that these same construction and agriculture companies were the most eager to contact hospital administration and ask to hire cheap Black patient-laborers. Over the decades, patients contributed to the groundskeeping crew, providing much of the labor to design and maintain large gardens in front of every building on campus.

Crownsville was not the only hospital in the world—or even in Maryland—that put its patients to work. Many asylums functioned like farm cooperatives, and doctors rightfully believed movement and time spent outdoors was beneficial to patients. Patient labor was often called industrial therapy, and it was popular in virtually every American mental hospital in the first half of the twentieth century. They often instituted factory-in-hospital programs, stealing inspiration from mental institutions that had long assigned patients tasks in England and Continental Europe. The goal was to institute work programs that would prepare patients for community placement and future vocations. Ideally, a patient's industrial therapy would develop through a gradient of employment from simple projects to complex training, and later to independent

employment in an industry. However, that's not what we find in Crownsville's records. Crownsville's patients helped to build their own hospital
with their bare hands and then contributed directly to the hospital's operation and budget. At the start, patients worked on less than 300 acres of
farmland. By 1939, 475 acres were under cultivation. By 1947, 550 acres
were under cultivation. In the late '50s, a superintendent told a grand
jury that approximately 600 Crownsville patients were engaged in unpaid
full- or part-time work on the farm or buildings. And by 1960, 700 acres
were under cultivation. In those early decades, the tasks provided patients
with little real-world training or contact. While some patients did find
employment, the hospital's own records did not describe that as the goal.

Photographs capture patients weaving rugs or tugging on willow
plants. The women worked in simple ankle-length dresses and the men
in overalls and white work shirts. The patients looked more like regular
field hands than sick patients—toiling outside in straw hats as they stood
beside mules, cows, and other livestock. This early dependency on Black
labor at the asylum was not unlike Southern plantations, and images

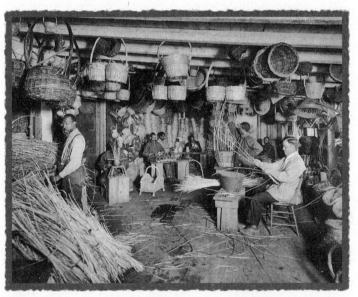

Many of the patients were talented basket weavers and artisans. Their work
was sold by the hospital to offset the cost of their own care, and often won
awards at local crafts shows. From the collections of the Maryland State
Archives.

show white nurses and doctors in the foreground supervising or even physically towering over their patients. In most photos the patients are seated. They often show staff staring directly into the camera, dominating the frame. There was little question about who held the power.

Historians of slavery and prisons have long argued that the commercial value of enslaved Black people in the American South was inextricably bound to their health status and their capacity to labor in the agricultural or domestic settings that had defined the Southern economy. Crownsville's founding took vestiges of chattel slavery—from the style of the rolls to the financial recordkeeping format used on plantations—and translated them to a clinical setting.

The twenty-fifth report of the Lunacy Commission included a financial report celebrating the savings Black patients provided to the state of Maryland. Officials described how patients with disabilities were assigned tasks that not only provided valuable labor but also allegedly made the patients less irritable.

William Murray, who was brutally murdered by a white employee at Crownsville, received a public eulogy that read more like a plaque for a hospital employee. The *Baltimore Afro-American*, a local newspaper for Black residents, wrote: "Mr. Murray had a good reputation for conduct

42   LUNACY COMMISSION OF

COMBINED STATEMENT SHOWING AGGREGATE SAVING ON FARM, CONSTRUCTION OF NEW BUILDINGS AND TEMPORARY QUARTERS BY THE UTILIZATION OF PATIENTS' EFFORTS.

Construction of new buildings..	$6,749 50
Estimation of farm labor..	2,317 80
Valuation of employment at temporary quarters.................	1,144 00
	$10,211 30
Deducting cost of maintaining patients employed for this work..	7,500 00
Saving to State by utilizing patients' labor.....................	$2,711 30
Net saving from operating farm....................................	7,167 68
Net saving from employing patients...............................	2,711 30
Total net saving...	$9,878 98

An image from the Twenty-Seventh Report of the Maryland Lunacy Commission of 1912. Government officials emphasized the costs saved through unpaid patient labor, and kept financial tables detailing costs, production timelines, and patient output.

and was employed in the rug shop. Often he turned out three or four small rugs a day which are sold by the institution for $3 a piece."

After his burial, William Murray's brother tried to submit a claim to the Industrial Accident Commission on the family's behalf, but the Murrays were denied because William was deemed not to be a real employee of the hospital. The institution had made three dollars apiece from his rugs but wouldn't have to pay his grieving family a dime.

Sadly, Murray was not alone in this regard. Patients at Crownsville were known for their exquisite craftsmanship and basket weaving, with their work often showcased at prestigious events such as the annual meeting of the American Psychological Association. But even as their art garnered accolades and prizes in cities like Baltimore, New Orleans, Phoenix, and Chicago, the patients' basic rights were ignored.

As I pored over the historical records of the first three decades of the hospital's existence, I was frustrated, but not surprised, by how challenging it was to unearth the medical information or personal stories of patients who had been relegated to the margins of society. Consistently, the records that did exist privileged the perspective of the state or the provider over the patient, who was almost never quoted or given the opportunity to speak for themselves. The files I managed to find often said so little and revealed so much at the same time. One particular record, dated March 28, 1938, encapsulated the mystery and heartbreak that surrounded this era. It described the admission of a toddler named Addie Belle Sellers, brought into Crownsville by a doctor named E. B. Iverson. The file had a simple heading: "Admission Note." Beneath it, the physician had penned a few brief lines about the child's condition:

This patient was carried in to this hospital to be admitted by Miss Little.

The child was clean and dressed in a blue snow suit. She is between twenty-seven months and three years of age and is not able to sit up alone. Her left eye has been removed, because of congenital cataract. She cried some while she was in the office and demonstrated a gross tremor of the arms.

She was carried to the ward and admitted as per routine.

The image of a three-year-old unable to sit upright was devastating. Reading the sparse details, I couldn't help but wonder about the circumstances that brought Addie Belle to Crownsville. What had become of her parents? How had she coped with loss and physical injury at such a young age? What had her life been like, and why was that information not part of her admission? I wanted to piece together fragments of the past and make them make sense. I had to accept that it was often impossible to fill in the blanks.

In those early years, the threat of death and disability was ever present on the grounds. Smallpox struck the patient wards in 1914 when a patient carrying the disease transferred to Crownsville from the county jail. Within six hours, staff leapt to vaccinate the entire patient population. Scarlet fever and diphtheria came, too.

During the tuberculosis outbreaks in the 1920s and '30s, the ramifications of the separation of Black patients at Crownsville became clear. While hospitals and asylums across the state were grappling with high death rates, Maryland's health department introduced a set of policies aimed at curbing the spread of tuberculosis. But the racial disparities that surfaced were impossible to ignore. Maryland had already made a point of prioritizing racial separation in the design of its hospital systems. When TB struck, white patients were organized by diagnosis and Black patients were organized by race. White patients at Springfield, Spring Grove, and Eastern Shore Hospitals were granted the privilege of isolated buildings where they could quarantine while still receiving mental healthcare. At first, there were no spare wards for quarantine at Crownsville—tuberculosis patients were housed alongside the general population. This exponentially increased Black patients' potential exposure to the disease and resulted in many deaths. But the explosion in cases eventually led hospital leaders to force the patients to build yet another building for themselves, this time a poorly constructed housing space for patients diagnosed with tuberculosis. The contrast in the treatment of the state's different patient populations was striking and underscored the deep-seated, race-based inequities that were woven into the fabric of the state's healthcare system.

By the 1930s, Crownsville Hospital's operations were hanging by a
thread. The institution, still under the leadership of Robert Winterode,
remained woefully understaffed twenty years into its existence. Those
first few dozen men had grown to a population of more than a thousand patients. The hospital had three physicians and a lone dentist on the
payroll, and was ill-equipped to handle the patients under its care and
the hundreds of new admissions it received each year. All of Maryland's
hospitals were inspected on a regular basis, but Crownsville's campus had
rapidly expanded. And with that growth came greater curiosity about
what was going on inside.

On a Thursday afternoon in April 1930, Superintendent Winterode
and his team welcomed a state employee and inspector named Alice Fitzgerald onto the grounds, and she set out to take notes on her findings.
Fitzgerald, a white woman with a professional nursing background, put
together a five-page summary on her typewriter, titled "Report of Visit of
Inspection of Crownsville State Hospital."

Entering Crownsville's grounds, Ms. Fitzgerald found the campus
quite beautiful. She appreciated the healing powers of a country setting,
and she looked out at the cluster of buildings and farmland, set back from
the road.

However, once behind its solid brick walls, she found a different story.
She noted that the female patients' wards were dreary and that the rooms
in which some of the "inmates" were locked were bare and depressing.
She wrote some reflections down, assuming that this dreariness was due
to a personnel shortage—and the fact that the personnel who were there
were not highly trained. The attendants were the lowest-paid and worked
the longest hours of all state employees.

"A patient must be locked in her cell-like room without even a bench
or rug to sit on because she is 'apt to wander' from the ward and there
is no one to watch her," she noted. There were only a few students and
attendants seen on duty. She wondered why the doors did not have small
slatted windows for easy patient supervision.

In the men's section of the hospital, she struggled to find someone in
charge. There were no male nurses around. "It is so easy to secure good

male nurses trained in psychiatry that it seems too bad to neglect securing them."

Thankfully, the beds and toilets on their side were clean and functional. The patients wore normal hospital gowns. She saw two patients sitting under a tarp inside continuous tubs. These tubs were one of the few early attempts at therapy, in which patients would sit for hours submerged in either scalding-hot or ice-cold water thought to calm their nerves. She found some temperature charts for patients who had been sent to the infirmary, and behavioral charts that were signed and well prepared. She noticed, however, that very few medicines were given.

She came across a large sewing room where a group of patients were working, but did not find much recreational space. In fact, she wrote, "Practically all the work in the institution is assigned to inmate help and must be very well supervised judging by good results."

Yet the nurses and attendants, living on two separate floors of shared employee housing, had closets, living rooms, studies, books, magazines, and a sun porch.

Fitzgerald concluded her report with great concern about the quality of the education and training provided to the employees, and with the goal to set up a nursing school at Crownsville. She urged state leaders to create some kind of recognition and a formal training degree, anything to make the job more attractive. After all that she had seen, she left that day most concerned about the prospects of the staff—not the patients.

A Family in the Forest

Outside the hospital walls and all along the Chesapeake Bay, the relationship between Black and white Marylanders, regardless of their mental status, was often defined by labor and power. In the same way that white doctors and lawmakers felt entitled to Black patients, white families at times felt entitled to their Black neighbors. These attitudes did not just loosely influence the hospital's practices and the possible biases of its early employees. They shaped lives and they changed family trajectories.

Gertrude Dorsey Belt was born in a tiny white concrete house in Annapolis on May 12, 1933, with the help of a midwife. Her parents raised her in a cabin in Sherwood Forest on the Severn River, the same river that a generation of enslaved people had fled to, where they climbed aboard ships to steal back their freedom in the middle of the night. The Sherwood Forest of Maryland is named after England's much more famous Sherwood Forest—the alleged home of the outlaw Robin Hood. Both woodlands are defined by inequality and a historical tension between the rich and the poor. But there would be no medieval hero swooping in to save anyone here.

Gertrude did what many poor Black girls had to do: she left school as a teenager and got to work cooking and cleaning for her white neighbors and trying to sell crafts. She had never seen crystal or cleaned silver before she stepped into their palatial homes. The cabins where she and her high school sweetheart, Freddy, lived often had only a tiny kitchen and no running water. Freddy would ride with Gertrude's father, Frank Dorsey, to help cut stones for builders in Washington, D.C. Frank would work such long and backbreaking hours that, eventually, Freddy would give up and hitchhike back home. Sometimes Gertrude and Freddy asked siblings or friends to feed their children and find space for them to sleep. They would come home from work with only enough to grab two pieces of bread and spread either butter or some old-school King Syrup from a can in between.

At eighteen, Gertrude and Freddy gave birth to a daughter they named Frederica. Then at nineteen, she had a son they named Fredrick. They expected their son would go on to be a stone cutter and builder like his father, and that their daughters would follow behind their mother into white Annapolitans' businesses and homes. But then Gertrude gave birth at age twenty to a wide-eyed, spirited baby in the private office of Dr. Aris T. Allen, his wife Dr. Faye Allen, and good friend Dr. Theodore Johnson, three Black physicians serving pregnant women at a time when they were still barred from the local white hospitals. Gertrude looked around the room, trying to figure out what to call this feisty girl. The couple had used Freddy's name enough times, so now it was Gertrude's turn. Gertrude passed on her own name and added Dr. Faye Allen's for good measure. Gertrude Faye Allen Belt was born on August 2, 1953. They called her Feefee and she was not going to follow the rules. Gertrude could sense it.

When I first spoke to Faye in April 2021, I had a feeling she was going to change this story. The first thing she wrote to me when I introduced myself was "OH MY GOD." She told me she had been waiting for someone to write about Crownsville. She had lost three loved ones in seven days in the midst of the Covid-19 pandemic, and many of the people who worked and lived at Crownsville would be transitioning soon, she told me. We were losing time.

A year and rounds of vaccinations later, in April 2022, I met Faye for the first time in person. I hopped in her brown Acura SUV, full of medical masks, sanitation wipes, and paperwork, and we rode all over Annapolis and Anne Arundel together. She took me to Crownsville Road. I'd been here before, but never with someone like her. She pointed to houses and told me where rows of corn or blackberry bushes once were, and where she used to play softball and break into the superintendent's private pool. For most of Faye's seventy years of life, Crownsville was everything. It was home. It was family. It became her mom's life work, and later, hers. "Boy, if this field could talk," she said with a laugh as we pulled up close to the administration building. "We used to tear them steps up."

Faye looked wistful as she surveyed the massive campus inspired by the Kirkbride architectural tradition, with many wings and passageways that sprung out from its center.

Weeds were sprouting on concrete steps. Windows had been smashed, and you could see through them that old beds, cabinets, and papers were lying out on cold hospital floors. There were rusty iron bars on the upper-level windows that would have once protected a patient from falling (or leaping) to their death. Paint had chipped and many floorboards had collapsed. Old lampposts were leaning down toward the earth. All across the campus, thick vines had broken through windows and were crawling up doorways and redbrick walls. The campus was a ghost town but, somehow, life seemed to be forcing its way through.

I looked at Faye and realized that this place had been its own universe.

I had been looking at Crownsville as an imposing place of study and investigation. She was looking at something more akin to a snow globe— a significant period of her life frozen in time and constrained in glass.

Only now the glass had been cracked. And covered in graffiti. At that time, the state, not the county, had ownership of Crownsville, and the campus was covered in signs that said Keep Out and No Trespassing. I asked her if we would get in trouble for driving up so close. "Oh yeah," she replied.

About seven minutes into our ride, a security patrol car pulled up to Faye. "No one is allowed on the property," the man explained. He leaned over to the window and politely asked us to leave. He looked exhausted. I was inclined to follow his rules. But Faye asked him, "Have you ever felt any of the energy on the property?"

His eyes lit up. He was gearing up to work his first-ever overnight shift alone in the dark. And lately, he explained, he'd been getting strange auras and sensations on the campus. Some of the more far-flung corners, near the old cottages and employee housing, frightened him. "I found out about the stuff that they used to do here at the hospital to Black people," he told us. "I felt a whole lot different then, all the rest of that day." He scratched at his arm and explained that his skin had been itching even though he had never had allergies before. "My skin just felt like it raised."

He looked at the two of us for a second and smiled. "You see that white truck right there? Why don't you pull up right there." Faye and I pulled over and parked.

We spent the next two hours with Paris, a Crownsville campus security officer and children's board game designer who lived near Indian Head, Maryland. I would find out firsthand why everyone thought Faye was different.

Paris seemed unable to stop pouring out his life story to her. Faye would listen, sometimes closing her eyes like she was breathing every detail about him in. He was working shifts at Crownsville and trying to make ends meet. He was having a hard time getting bookstores and local gift shops to review his latest board games and give him a shot. He had a vision for a series of children's games and books that explored Black history, pride, and mental health. "I really kind of lost my fire," he told her, his eyes welling up with tears. He felt like he had gone backward.

There was also pressure in his personal life. A member of his family was struggling with depression and anxiety, and he couldn't find a Black doctor or psych nurse to work with them. He told Faye that he was tired of their insurance sending them to white doctors who didn't understand their life experiences. She nodded knowingly. Faye gave him her number and the name of a Black doctor she would call on his behalf in their area. She told him he had nothing to be embarrassed about. He was taking care of himself and his family the best way he knew how, and this would all be part of the story one day.

"It's funny, I'm telling you, I just was saying to myself that I needed some inspiration for me to get back," he replied through tears. He thanked her profusely for being kind and listening to someone she had only just met. For the rest of the afternoon, the three of us explored Crownsville together. Paris looked like he was floating, light on his feet.

In her earliest memories, Faye says she was seeing colors. Later, she learned to call them auras. They started out as flashing lights, deep reds and pinks in the forest where she used to play. She thought they were sunbeams dancing between the leaves for the last time before the day gave way to night. But as time passed, the colors grew more vibrant, their presence stronger. They would dazzle and pulse with a life of their own. They would hover over the people in her life, wrapping them in a warmth that drew her in or a chill that would repulse her.

Faye had no idea what was happening to her. She only knew that she was different, that there was something unique about her perception of the world. Her mother, Gertrude, was baffled by her daughter's strange behavior at times. Faye could get lost in her own thoughts, caught up in the colors swirling around her.

By elementary school, Faye realized only she could see them. She panicked. Classmates would say, "*Feefee*, you're crazy." At night, she prayed to God that this strange gift would leave her be. But it stuck and only grew stronger. Faye started to believe that the colors carried meaning. A warning of something to come. An indication of someone's intentions.

She was a "tomboy" who played baseball with the boys and ran wild behind her parents' one-bedroom wooden shack. She knew she was poor—her mother had told her as much—but in the outdoors Faye was convinced she was lucky and free.

Everywhere else seemed to remind her that Black girls had to grow up fast—that there was a predetermined path leading to a life of servitude. Most of the Black people she knew worked in the kinds of jobs that had them pushing brooms with little protection. The only people she knew with "nice things" were white. The family's cabin sat just outside the gates and brick walls that protected big, beautiful homes of Sherwood Forest. Whenever they were together in downtown Annapolis, Gertrude would ask her three kids to toss coins into fountains and make a wish for a "real" home.

When her mother eventually encouraged her to take her first job as a domestic worker before her eighth birthday, Faye didn't resist. She agreed to work for a wealthy white family that lived down the road. She didn't have much of a choice in the matter.

The family she worked for had three toddlers and a long list of tasks for her to manage: wash the clothes, press the husband's shirts for work, cook for the family, clean the house, and entertain the children. One child was older and independent, one toddler would sprint around the house, and one would stare up at Faye and demand to be carried everywhere. Faye didn't like the feeling, the aura around their home.

Faye remembers the children's mother walking out, leaving her feeling desperate and alone. Faye looked around, grabbed all the laundry and the husband's old work shirts, and threw everything she could into a bin. She scooped up the three kids and dragged them next door to another white family's home. Faye banged on the door. Before they could protest, she shouted, "Here, you take 'em."

Faye sauntered home. She knew she was about to get an earful, and the weight of her decision settled into her bones. She listened to the apple trees shake and the leaves crunch under her feet. Sherwood Forest had always been her comfort. It seemed to want to reassure her that she could walk another path.

Sure enough, her former boss drove right up to Gertrude and Freddy's home in the sleekest car Faye had ever seen. Faye stood there in the yard with her hands on her hips, waiting for the inevitable, watching as the woman stomped on their grass and demanded to speak to Gertrude.

"You have no idea what your child has done," the woman spat. To Faye's surprise, Gertrude remained calm. "Miss, I know my baby. If she doesn't want to work for you, she won't."

The woman sped off in her garish car. Faye and Gertrude stood several feet apart, staring at each other.

"Mama," Faye shouted, "I'm not going to be like you! I'm not going to work for these white people. I'm going to be somebody."

Faye spoke something into her own life and her mother's. Already, Gertrude was on the path to becoming a nurse and building her own career. Her daughter would one day follow behind. They would make their way out of the forest, away from neighbors who viewed them as little more than a cheap and convenient labor source.

The conditions for Black families in Maryland in the first half of the twentieth century were a painful limitation and a catalyst all at once. The expectations of their white neighbors were an insult to their abilities but also a foreshadowing of what would happen as Black people—and Black patients—continued to demand more for themselves in Annapolis. The Belt family and many others would arrive in spaces like Crownsville and transform them. They would fight on behalf of patients, investigate their mistreatment, and ask for the government and the community to do more for them. Sometimes they would win. Often, they would lose.

They would find themselves back in familiar patterns—working for white doctors and administrators, struggling to be heard and respected, and pressing up against a ceiling of possibility. Still, Crownsville Hospital would bring mother and daughter together. It was the rejection of the status quo, the possibility of a life outside of servitude that changed the Belt family and others for generations to come. Faye may have ended up a bit like her mama. Or her mama turned out to be more like her than she ever imagined.

CHAPTER 4

What Could Drive a Black Person Mad?

I N THE 1930S, NEARLY A HUNDRED MILES SEPARATED TWO MEN, MAT- thew Williams and George Armwood, from Anne Arundel County. Their families didn't have the right words for it then, but both men were considered strange and "different" from birth. Had they lived on another shore, their paths very likely could have led them to the doors of Crownsville Hospital.

But Williams and Armwood called the Eastern Shore home. And both men's lives came to an end hanging from a tree.

For Black people living in Annapolis and Baltimore, a disability or emotional disorder could lead to warehousing and confinement at Crownsville or a county jail. But on the Eastern Shore, Black men seen as cognitively impaired were subjected to something different: indentured servitude.

For generations, the Eastern Shore was notorious for its reliance on indentured servitude and slavery. It was part of the proud social fabric, and it supported the entire agricultural economy and way of life. Long before the Chesapeake Bay Bridge united the agricultural and fishing communities of the Eastern Shore with the bustling Western Shore, towns like Princess Anne, Crisfield, Deal Island, and Salisbury were more remote and rural than they are today. The area is one of the oldest American communities, with most of its inhabitants tracing their roots back to colonial migrations from England and Ireland in the seventeenth and eighteenth centuries. In the wake of emancipation, the status of Black people changed in Maryland's Eastern Shore as it did across the United States.

Continued indentured servitude was something of an open secret, and not just on the Eastern Shore. In 1927 a grand jury report found that an institute called the House of Reformation for Colored Boys in southern Maryland was forcing young Black boys to work on local farms and in businesses like broom factories. The school was intended to "instruct" and "reform" boys who had been labeled as vicious and improper, and many of the boys housed there were known to be "mentally deficient." The investigators found that the boys were being farmed out in direct competition with regular laborers, and that, in many cases, they weren't receiving proper food and care. The investigators were especially concerned about the boys put to work in the broom shop, which was full of dust and flammable material and called a "menace to the life and health" of the boys. It was slavery by another name. In the report they wrote that "apparently no industrial training of any value is provided, and a boy on leaving the institution, is almost or quite as unfitted to face the world as he was when he was committed."

The Eastern Shore fought aggressively to maintain this kind of system—and for decades after slavery's end, Black people continued to serve as the cheap labor source on the region's farms. As a result, Black families lived in desperate poverty, and they would sometimes give away their children, especially those with developmental disabilities, to white families looking for a laborer or maid. These children effectively became slaves again.

Matthew "Buddie" Williams found himself trapped in this system. Williams had known hardship from an early age, after losing his mother to pneumonia when he was just four years old and then his father at age eight. He was taken in by his aunt and uncle in the Black district of Salisbury, Maryland. Newspaper records and old interviews with his relatives suggest that Matthew had a cognitive impairment—described as a "subnormality"—that made it hard for him to relate to others and to read emotion. Despite his disability, friends said that Williams valued honesty and hard work. Even so, he was viewed by both Black and white residents as "demented" and unworthy of a regular salary.

He took a job helping a wealthy man named Daniel J. Elliott. For seven or eight years, Williams toiled in Elliott's box factory and lumber-yard for $1.50 per day, often doing additional work for Elliott's family on the side.

On December 4, 1931, eighteen-year-old Matthew Williams went to work as he always did. But on this cold Friday afternoon, he was upset as he entered Elliott's office on Lake Street wanting to discuss his low wages. He found Elliott on the phone with another prominent Salisbury businessman, Thomas Chatham.

From the other end of the phone, Chatham heard two gunshots and called the authorities. The police found a mysterious scene: D. J. Elliott dead at his desk, Mr. Elliott's son, James, alive in the room, and Matthew Williams shot several times but still alive.

James Elliott took control of the narrative. He claimed that he heard shots from the house and ran in to find his father dead and Williams covered in blood. He said that as he left to go find help, Williams tried to flee. To stop him, James shot him in the shoulder and the leg.

But another rumor spread on the Black side of town. Matthew Williams hadn't fought with his boss about low pay. He had lent James Elliott a sum of money that he had saved on condition that the money would be returned. When attempts by Williams to get repaid by the younger Elliott failed, Williams tried to take the matter up with the older Elliott. James walked into their meeting, rumor had it, and shot both Williams and his own father.

What really happened remains a mystery. As a Black man with a cognitive disability, Matthew Williams never stood a chance. The crowd made sure he never had an opportunity to tell his story.

Williams arrived at Peninsula General Hospital semiconscious and bleeding out from his wounds. The hospital staff quickly formed a judgment. Williams, already labeled as strange, was restrained in a strait-jacket to keep him from being violent.

The *Salisbury Times* mistakenly reported that Williams died at the hospital, but as soon as they learned he was still alive, around 7:30 p.m. that night, a sign was posted on the *Salisbury Times* building correcting their previous statement. People left work and closed up shops to join a growing mob.

A group entered the hospital, demanding that Williams be turned over to them. They were stopped by Police Chief N. H. Holland and Deputy John Parks, who blocked the entrance. Six members of the mob then went around the building to an open side entrance and reached the Negro ward. Unsurprisingly, this section wasn't well protected. There, hospital superintendent Helen V. Wise surrendered: "If you must take him, do it quietly."

The men threw Williams, covered in bandages and wearing a straitjacket, out of a hospital window and into the crowd of three hundred people waiting below.

As men carried Williams to the courthouse, the crowd swelled, until a mob of some thousand people surrounded Williams. He was pushed, stabbed with an ice pick, and dragged by a truck. County Sheriff Phillips attempted to prevent the lynching, but the mob pushed him to the side.

At 8:00 p.m., the crowd fixed up a noose and found a branch twenty feet above the ground. They tied an unconscious Williams by the neck and began to lift him up, then drop him down. Over and over again. The mob allowed Williams to hang lifelessly for twenty minutes, as they mocked the victim and took parts of his anatomy as souvenirs.

After Williams thumped to the ground one last time, the crowd followed the body as it was dragged behind a truck once again, this time toward the Black section of Salisbury off Poplar Hill Avenue. Finally, after about an hour of further torture of his corpse, Williams was tied to a lamppost, doused in gasoline and oil, and set on fire in front of a store so, as the papers reported, "all the colored people could see him." According to local Black reporters with the *Afro*, Black residents, fleeing in terror, could smell Matthew Williams's burning flesh in the air. The mob removed Williams's fingers and toes and threw them on the porches of Black homes, shouting that they should make nigger sandwiches.

The sheriff eventually recovered Matthew Williams's body from the tired, drunken mob, and cut it down from the lamppost. He dumped the body in a field outside of town.

The Williams family, heartbroken, wanted the body back for a proper burial. The Black undertaker, James Stewart, took it upon himself to recover the body from the field and brought it back for a funeral, which was held at Stewart's Funeral Home in Salisbury.

Some argue that Matthew Williams's lynching was, at least in part, in response to the delayed "justice" the Eastern Shore experienced the previous year with the trial of Euel Lee, aka Orphan Jones, accused of murdering a white family of four in Berlin, Maryland. Lee's lawyer, Bernard Ades, felt that there was no way he would receive a fair trial on the Eastern Shore and had the hearing moved to Baltimore, which deeply angered the residents of Worcester County and the Delmarva Peninsula as a whole. The Euel Lee case dragged on for two years as the NAACP and the Urban League fought tooth and nail for a fair trial. The residents of the Eastern Shore wanted swift justice to control the Black population; aggressive lawyers and big-city jails to protect Black men were simply unacceptable.

Because of Euel Lee, and because of the Eastern Shore's violent history of taking the law into its own hands, lynch law was effectively a legitimate form of power. Lawyers, due process, and city jurors would have no role in the system that meted out justice to alleged Black criminals on the Eastern Shore.

Immediately after hearing of the Williams lynching in Salisbury, Governor Albert C. Ritchie set up a task force with Attorney General William P. Lane Jr. to look into prosecuting those who were involved with the mob. After interviewing police officers and hospital workers who were present during the abduction, they found that no one could recall or recognize any of the thousands of people that were present that night. To this day, almost a hundred years later, no one has been prosecuted for the lynching of Matthew Williams.

The white journalist H. L. Mencken fiercely attacked the Eastern Shore in the *Baltimore Sun*, calling it an "Alsatia of morons" where social degeneration had allowed "ninth-rate men" to come to power. Following

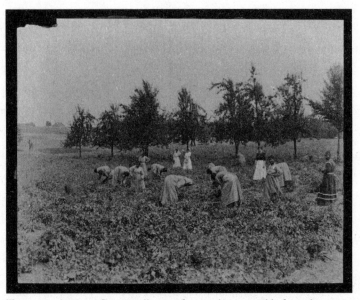

The women living at Crownsville were frequently responsible for picking pro-duce and tending to the fields and gardens. Many patients descended from the Eastern Shore, and would have been familiar with agricultural practices. They were not paid. Some records suggest the patients enjoyed the fresh air and distraction. From the collections of the Maryland State Archives.

the article, Salisbury merchants canceled $150,000-worth of business from Baltimore firms that advertised in the paper.

George Armwood lived his whole life on the Eastern Shore. He considered himself a hard worker and by all accounts was eager to find his place in the world, despite an undiagnosed mental disability that left him something of an outcast.

When a white, prominent, and powerful local businessman approached Armwood's mother to take George out of school so he could work, she readily agreed. By 1931, he was employed by Mr. John H. Richardson, under an arrangement that prevented George from being committed to a psychiatric facility. He had a reputation for being a good worker, but with a "feeble mind": George was known to be "off at times," but always put his head down and worked hard to make a meaningful life for himself.

George and John had a good relationship and respected each other.

Richardson was a tall and lanky farmer, and George was young and strong. So good was their relationship that in the summer of 1933, they concocted a plan to make some quick cash.

The two decided to rob Mrs. Mary Denston, a local seventy-one-year-old white woman, as she was known to carry large sums of money on herself as she walked alone on the dirt road that connected her house to her daughter's farm. It was supposed to be simple: Armwood would hide in the woods until Mrs. Denston passed, then he'd jump out, grab the money, and run. Richardson and Armwood would divide the loot and no one would be the wiser.

After the robbery, employees of the State Roads Commission found Mrs. Denston by the side of the road, in shock. They took her to Sheriff Luther Daugherty and she reported the assault to police in Somerset County. The force organized a search party to look for Armwood in the woods nearby.

A mob turned rumors of a robbery into a story of rape. That fiction gave way to something even stranger: residents heard that Armwood had chewed off both of Mrs. Denston's breasts. The *Salisbury Times* wrote: "Mrs. Denston was reported to be in a critical condition from shock but was able to give officers a description of the assailant, who, she described as a short 'strange' negro."

The police questioned witnesses in the area and searched the home of Armwood's mother, Etta, in Manokoo. But George Armwood was found hiding in the home of his employer, John H. Richardson. The police dragged him across a field and beat him as he was taken into custody. Etta told reporters from the *Afro-American* newspaper that she feared the police would kill her son. Armwood signed a confession under the watch of state police after being questioned by Lieutenant Ruxton Ridgely.

John Richardson, the man who came up with the original scheme, was taken to jail after the crime, held for a month, and then released after claiming he had no knowledge of what happened.

Police took Armwood to Salisbury prison, ten miles north of Princess Anne. They hoped the distance would keep potential lynchers at bay. Within three minutes of his arrival at Salisbury prison, a rapidly growing crowd appeared. State police called the governor to inform him they would move Armwood for fear of mob violence. They made a request to place him in the Baltimore City Jail and brought him over there before the request was even approved or denied.

The police sought distance to protect Armwood because, just two years earlier, the lynching of Matthew Williams had embarrassed the state of Maryland and given the Eastern Shore a "lynchtown" reputation.

However, Maryland's powerful political players stepped in and decided Armwood's fate. Somerset County judge Robert F. Duer and State Attorney John B. Robins were pressured by locals and called for Armwood's return to the Eastern Shore. The two assured Governor Ritchie that justice would not be circumvented by terror and lynch law. They said Armwood would be safe in Princess Anne. Governor Ritchie relented, and Armwood was sent back to Princess Anne in the early morning of October 17. Twenty-five state police escorted Armwood.

Despite the promises made by Duer and Robins, the mob returned—this time in larger numbers. Judge Duer drove to the scene while he was on his way to a dinner party. He stopped in front of the crowd and addressed them. "I know nearly all of you," he said. He pleaded that he was "one of them" and would hold the citizens "to their honor." The crowd dispersed, but it quickly reassembled, nearing two thousand. Members of the mob hurled bricks at the police.

Deputy Norman Dryden, Captain Edward McKim Johnson, and twenty-three other officers guarding the jailhouse threw tear gas at the mob. As the smoke cleared, the lynch mob used two fifteen-foot timbers as battering rams to breach the jailhouse doors. Captain Johnson was reportedly knocked unconscious. Deputy Dryden gave in and simply handed over the keys to the mob.

The mob, now consisting of five thousand men, women, and children, found Armwood hiding under his mattress. They dragged him from the cell and placed a noose around his neck. They beat him, stabbed and kicked him, tied him to the back of a truck, and drove him to a tree on the property of ninety-one-year-old Thomas Bock. The crowd had initially planned to take him to Duer's home, but changed course. Before hanging him, they cut off Armwood's ears and ripped teeth from his jaw. Some reported that Armwood was already dead from the beatings before he was strung up from a tree branch. His body had been dragged for a mile.

The lynchers then dragged George Armwood's corpse back to the courthouse in downtown Princess Anne. They hung his body from a telephone pole and burned it. Around midnight, a garbage truck hauled George Armwood's corpse to Hayman's Lumber Yard. Fearing for his life, the town's Black undertaker refused to take charge of the body. The state police intervened and arranged to have it buried among local Black families.

State leaders blamed Judge Duer and State Attorney Robins for Armwood's lynching and opened an investigation to identify members of the mob. Somerset residents refused to inform on their neighbors. One sheriff allegedly said, "I did not see a single man from Somerset County in the bunch."

The investigation included a grand jury convened to hear testimony from forty-two witnesses to the Armwood lynching. The people of Princess Anne and the Eastern Shore protected each other. Those interviewed claimed that the organizers of the lynching were not from the local community and that they could not identify a single person involved.

However, Ralph Matthews, editor of the *Afro-American* newspaper, interviewed law enforcement and residents. It was clear that many people of Salisbury and Princess Anne were deeply involved with the lynching and the police knew who they were. Duer knew that the mob was not composed of strangers and out-of-towners, but locals, and some well-connected community members. The people of the Eastern Shore were proud to be "lynchtown." At least in private.

State police ultimately identified nine men as leaders of the mob that lynched George Armwood. Attorney General Preston Lane sent a letter to the state's attorney John B. Robins listing the names, addresses, and occupations of the nine participants. Robins dragged his feet.

On Tuesday, November 28, 1933, suspects in the George Armwood lynching were arrested by the National Guard in Salisbury.

When the National Guard arrived, hostilities between the locals and the Guard spilled into the public eye as news spread of the Guard's purpose in Princess Anne. It reached the point where local chants of "Lynch Lane" prompted the state attorney general to leave the city. The grand jury declined to indict anyone. One thousand white supporters cheered as the accused were released. There were no further efforts to prosecute anyone for George Armwood's murder.

A year later, in 1934, the Senate Judiciary Committee opened a probe into lynchings in the United States and the persistent failure of local governments to stop them. The Senate invited Preston Lane to speak as a witness to the George Armwood lynching. Lane provided eight names of men involved in the lynching that he had personally observed, and the men's names were published in newspapers. However, Congress and the federal courts had no jurisdiction to act, and because the grand jury did not indict, the case was closed. One of the named participants, William H. Thompson, appeared before the Senate to assert his innocence, claiming he was not even in Princess Anne at the time.

The function of lynching was so much more than a bypassing of the justice system. It was a form of psychological terrorism. And it sent several messages. One basic message was that they had killed people like Williams and Armwood before and, if necessary, would do it again.

But the more subtle and crucial message was that they still owned Black people. That they could sever their body parts, and continue to have complete and utter dominion. They controlled their livelihoods and their prospects. They could take ownership of people seen as destitute, different, and strange. They also owned the narrative. Each lynching stole the life of its victim, but it also wrought immeasurable trauma on every Black person who witnessed or heard the story.

Between 1889 and 1930, 3,724 people were lynched in the South; over four-fifths were Black. In almost every case, no serious effort was made to identify and punish lynchers.

How could you not go mad?

CHAPTER 5

The Architecture of Injustice

O N A SNOWY WINTER WEEKEND IN FEBRUARY 2015, I GRABBED MY warmest coat, stuffed several notebooks and manila folders into a ragged L.L.Bean backpack, and flew from Boston's Logan Airport to Baltimore. I was on my way to the Maryland State Archives for the very first time. I had completed ethics training and made an official request through the Department of Health and Mental Hygiene. After months of back-and-forth with government officials, I had been granted access to a trove of records that even some former employees of Crownsville Hospital couldn't see. I was about to delve into the complex history of the asylum, through historical photographs, administrative notes, meeting minutes, interview transcripts, and other key records that would illuminate what Crownsville meant to the thousands of people who called it home for much of their lives.

I took a cab into Annapolis and sought out a man named Paul Lurz. Paul is a former Crownsville staff member and is well known to local historians and archivists. The legend I'd heard was that Paul had almost singlehandedly rescued and preserved the history of Crownsville Hospital. In the final months before the hospital closed in 2004, Paul made split-second decisions that changed everything. He had found crucial material, like the hospital's autopsy records, infested with insects and abandoned in a basement. He gathered them and organized them into locked and fireproof filing cabinets in his personal office in the administration building. When the state shuttered the hospital in 2004, the Maryland State Archives were able to build their collection thanks to Paul.

I'd already interviewed Paul extensively over the phone in the preceding months, but that morning we were reconnecting in person over coffee and bagels so he could ready me for what I might uncover in the archives. Some of the archivists at the Maryland State Archives and employees in Mental Hygiene had not been able to tell me much about what I would be able to access—I could barely get some of them to answer the phone. But one archives employee and close friend of Paul Lurz, a historian named Rob Schoeberlein, had been incredibly helpful and enthusiastic about my desire to learn more about Crownsville and the treatment of Black patients. It became clear to me that Paul and Rob had led much of this preservation effort on their own, and that they had a special interest in the hospital and its patients that was not necessarily shared by the rest of the state.

Around ten that morning, Paul and I sat across from each other at a bagel shop. I thanked him profusely for spending dozens of hours with me on the phone. I tried to pay for his food but he wouldn't let me. Secretly, I was grateful. I had no money and had funded parts of my research and meals by taking part in a series of psychology and neurology studies at Harvard, letting people prod and quiz me so I could get some quick cash. He shrugged off my thank-yous like it had all been nothing, and pulled out a new folder of some photographs he had found since we last spoke. We mostly sat in silence, as decades of life on Crownsville's campus unfolded before us. I glanced up and noticed Paul looked sorrowful. He was gazing at an old photograph of children gathered on the hospital's lawn. Paul, who had worked with children and administration at Crownsville for forty years, had dedicated his entire life to the hospital. It dawned on me just how intricate daily operations must have been at an asylum of that size, and how many individuals must have lived and toiled in its halls before it suddenly shut down. I recognized that even in the face of an institution's failures or harm, there were individuals like

Paul who showed up every single day with a commitment to doing a lot of good.

Paul wished me luck and we said our goodbyes. I left feeling anxious, knowing that I was new to the messy work of sifting through archives. I walked up to the archives' front doors and stepped up to a counter. I handed over my signed permission forms, confidentiality agreements, and letters of recommendation from my professors. An employee behind the desk reminded me that very few had ever received access to the boxes she was about to pull.

I settled down at a simple library table. A moment later, an archivist brought over a series of archival document boxes or "clamshells." Paul had warned me that it might be overwhelming at first. It was.

For the next several hours, I took meticulous notes. I found myself frustrated at just how much was left out by the original doctors and recordkeepers. In some boxes there were stacks of index cards bearing patient records, but those cards were mostly empty, with little beyond the patient's name and the signature of the supervising physician. Very few even documented a conclusive diagnosis, and of those that did, the prognosis was limited to a short phrase lacking context or a treatment plan. I found myself wondering who these records were really for. If a physician needed to pick up where another left off, how would they have found the information they needed to treat someone? If a patient was being discharged, would they or their loved ones have an accurate history of the treatments and interventions that had worked or failed? Later, I found out that decades of patient records had been destroyed in the early 1960s.

I was sifting through the records of an institution that had since been shut down, hoping that the documents left behind might speak for the people no longer able to. Instead, I learned a great deal about the patients' homemade products and how much it cost the state to house them—and a whole lot about state leaders and administrators in the early twentieth century who were clearly worried about the hospital's budget, future, and reputation in a segregated state. Later, I found evidence of a Black community becoming increasingly aware throughout the first half of the twentieth century that at Crownsville, something had gone very wrong.

Separate and Unequal

In July 1943, Randall Tyus, executive secretary of the Baltimore chapter of the NAACP, wrote an urgent memorandum to the governor and Maryland's Interracial Commission. Just a few days prior, on June 30, Tyus and a group of concerned Black citizens had visited Crownsville State Hospital. The men were given only a short period of time to explore the hospital, and were trailed by Superintendent Winterode and other top administrators. With Tyus was local Reverend Hiram Smith, and Dr. J.E.T. Camper, who was critical of Crownsville and who suspected that patients were being exploited.

What they discovered left the men distraught. The white attendants had no education and no training. In their short visit, they took note of three different patients showing multiple head and facial injuries. In each case, Dr. Winterode's team insisted the patient had simply fallen. One patient called out to Tyus and his companions as they were leaving, begging them to get him out. He feared the guards would kill him.

The three men found that there was no recreational equipment for patients. The outdoor recreation space that did exist was limited to a small, fenced-in area full of trees that hadn't been cleared for any kind of activity.

Housed among the regular population were men who had been transferred to the hospital from the city jail and were allegedly criminally insane. There were detention cells, but with none of the proper hospital equipment. The young children housed at Crownsville were receiving no form of schooling or job training whatsoever. And there were widespread reports that some of the patients were being used "in abnormal ways sexually."

Dr. Camper met with a patient named Doris Dotson, a Black woman born in Brooklyn, Maryland. She had been a student at the Hampton Institute in Virginia and had been referred to Johns Hopkins for a mental health evaluation. They sent her to Crownsville. The hospital had labeled her troublesome. Staff threw her into a cell with no clothes on and poured cold water on her. As Dr. Camper visited with Doris, he realized that a visibly disturbed patient had been placed in charge of her care—instead of one of the hospital's employees. He then observed that the women on her ward were being bathed by the male patients as punishment for any violent behavior.

Tyus received a phone call at the NAACP offices. A mother, Mrs. Geneva Taylor, wanted their help in securing the freedom of her son, Melvin. Melvin had been working in a local war plant and had been struck in the head by a piece of equipment. Mrs. Taylor was desperate, insisting to the doctor that her son was perfectly fine. She suspected that he was being held at Crownsville because the company he worked for was worried that if he was pronounced sane and released, his testimony might prove them liable for his injuries and increase the damages the family could receive.

Finally, the trio met with a white man and employee named Joseph Muller, who had started working at the hospital on May 4, 1943, a couple of months before the visit. Muller told the men that the patients were given rotten food and forced to sleep on bare floors. Many of his colleagues and fellow attendants would sleep on the job, drink, and play cards. They routinely beat the patients almost to death. Mr. Muller claimed that two patients that he knew had died after receiving these beatings. Muller was clearly shaken; he had been an attendant in white hospitals for over thirty years, but the conditions at Crownsville were by far the worst he'd ever experienced. By May 17, 1943, Muller had seen enough. He quit.

His final act was to confront a supervisor and tell him the truth of what was happening to the hospital's patients. The man allegedly scoffed, "To hell with the Niggers."

The Worst Story Ever Told

Throughout the first half of the twentieth century, the records paint a very clear picture. The conditions at Crownsville were violent and exploitative. For the first several decades, racial hierarchy and state-sanctioned segregation ensured the hospital's all-white staff dominated their patients and controlled the official narratives of what was happening. In response, a community of Black residents working with the NAACP and the families of patients started to raise alarms.

Their volunteer efforts, and the letters and notes they wrote, were crucial not only to the future of patient care, but to correcting a whitewashed record of the hospital's operations. Black church groups and women's clubs were among the first to come and visit Crownsville's patients. It wasn't until 1954, though, that African American community leaders decided to step up and create the Crownsville Auxiliary, which welcomed both Black and white female volunteers. I spent time talking to Essie Sutton, a dressmaker from West Baltimore, who was one of those dedicated volunteers. She passed away at the age of ninety-seven in 2021. She spent more than four decades helping out at the hospital. One of her first observations was that many of the hospital's patients seemed just like "you or me." She even recognized a few of them from her own neighborhood. She wasn't a nurse or doctor, but it seemed to her that, in some cases, "they should've been at home."

Essie was proud to have planned fun events like dances and parties for the patients, but especially cherished the opportunity to establish a canteen where patients could buy sandwiches, coffee, candy, cigarettes. These were small but powerful acts that brought joy and humanity to an otherwise bleak environment.

But in those early years, the network of volunteers could not outweigh the hospital's white employees, who weren't always as committed to humane care. They held deeply ingrained biases that Black people were more prone to aggression and more responsive to punitive, carceral tactics. The staff at Crownsville leaned heavily on seclusion as a primary method for subduing patients. Patients at Crownsville were routinely left alone in dark and damp cells with little more than a thin mattress on the ground.

The practice of isolating and secluding patients was well documented and, in some instances, critiqued. In 1949, a document titled "Report on the Mental Hospitals of the State of Maryland" expressed concern that recreation had still not been developed at Crownsville and that the few amusements offered to the patients came from volunteers from the

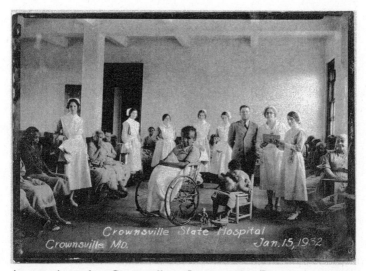

A women's ward at Crownsville in January 1932. During this period, patients living with developmental differences and mental health diagnoses, as well as children who had become orphaned would all live together in crowded wards. They spent much of the day seated in bare rooms like this one. From the collections of the Maryland State Archives.

community. Furthermore, officials wrote, "restraints by means of camisoles, wristlets, and anklets [were] used sparingly" while "seclusion [was] more freely used and civil patients [were] secluded in the section for that purpose on the criminal ward."

The staff allegedly passed over the first-line tools and practices of restraint and resorted to patient seclusion and confinement. The 1949 report suggested that this practice was an inappropriate and severe form of care for the average patient, who did not need to be kept in isolation cells meant for the small population of patients who had committed crimes. In those early years, less than 5 percent of patients had any sort of criminal record. So, although a small fraction of Crownsville patients entered the asylum classified as dangerous, the employees at Crownsville were alleged to be engaging in an unusual preference for confinement and seclusion.

These were not minor custodial issues that frustrated the occasional employee, but rather attention-grabbing features of hospital order. The rumors about the use of seclusion cells and rampant, racist physical abuse began to spread around the state. Reporters started sniffing around the hospital. And in 1949, one Pulitzer Prize–winning, Washington-based reporter by the name of Howard Norton managed to get unfettered access to Crownsville State Hospital and the rest of the state's system. Built to hold six thousand people, the system was currently housing nine thousand in deplorable circumstances. Historian Jonathan Engel put it plainly: "The hospitals were breeding mental illness faster than they were curing it."

In January 1949, after Norton had completed his tour of Crownsville, the title of his investigative series read, "Maryland's Shame: The Worst Story Ever Told in the Sunpapers."

Norton had discovered that Crownsville, the only place—public or private—willing to take in Black residents, had only eight doctors to take care of more than 1,800 men, women, and children, whom he described as being "herded into its buildings."

"Crownsville is supposed to do for Negro children what Rosewood Training School supposedly does for feeble-minded white children. But there is *no school* at Crownsville."

Men and women were sleeping in basement storage rooms and in sweltering attics without fire escapes. Children were two to a bed, sleeping feet-to-head. Some were overflowing out onto porches and going to sleep in rooms that had been designated for recreation. Children shared space with men who had been labeled as sex offenders.

The hospital was struggling in large part because it was having more trouble attracting white prospective employees than the other state hospitals, and the state was offering them dismal pay. The result was a shocking ratio of one doctor per 225 patients, and a hospital that was only occasionally offering psychotherapy. Furthermore, the hospital had only 110 attendants, though its budget allowed for 217.

And seclusion for patients was not always just a dirty empty room or an overcrowded porch; the conditions in secluded areas of Crownsville were often brutal and subhuman. In notes from the Mental Hygiene Board of Review's meeting to discuss Crownsville in March 1954—more than a half decade after Norton's exposé—board members discussed an area of the hospital commonly called "the cage." The board described the cage as being a well-known isolated area for disturbed female patients. Hospital staff were keeping eighty women there, despite having sleeping space for only thirty-five. In addition to the overcrowding, employees wrote that there was "a very serious shortage of water, both for drinking and bathing in this part of the hospital" and that the staff had not yet been able to relieve the overcrowding or water deficiencies.

While white institutions such as Springfield Hospital also experienced crisis-level overcrowding and filth during the first half of the twentieth century, the physical spaces were rarely described in as desperate terms. Springfield had originally been built as a summer home and slave plantation. It was stately and well resourced by comparison to Crownsville, and its patients enjoyed the benefits of a nearby well-connected public transportation line.

At Crownsville, seclusion was common and conditions were recognized by hospital workers as inhospitable and cruel. And yet the same cells and patterns of abuse persisted for years. The abnormal treatment of Crownsville's patients did not go unnoticed at the time, as they often festered in plain view of attendants and inert officials. It was only with the help of civil rights activists, Black doctors, and reporters—and in spite of state leaders—that patients' stories occasionally pushed past hospital walls.

Why Was Less Being Done?

Paul Lurz has been my pen pal for ten years. He's taken on the role of a surrogate grandparent, sharing some of my NBC News reports on his Facebook page like he had a hand in raising me. He sends me emails asking me how my loved one is responding to medication. At times, he has reminded me to go enjoy the outdoors, and he lets me know when his flowers are about to bloom. Whenever I'm in Annapolis he invites me to have coffee and to try his fresh, homemade fig jam. We've created our own unexpected bond, swapping research, photographs, questions, and stories about a little-known Jim Crow asylum.

Paul is gentle and kind. He has a long white beard, and he likes to tug on it as though that'll help pull out the deepest and most buried memories. He sort of looks like a tall and lean Santa Claus. He's from Baltimore City, but he's a country boy at heart. An enduring joy throughout his time at Crownsville was having free rein to explore the grounds.

Paul was born in the 1940s in a row house in the Brewers Hill neighborhood, a community named after the breweries founded by German immigrants. Some of his earliest childhood memories are strangely punctuated by the smell of beer.

When Paul was nine years old, he heard a commotion and the sirens of police cars outside. His neighbor, Ms. Mary, beloved by all the children in the neighborhood, was outside, shouting. Her husband had called the police and asked them to take her to an asylum. The local housewives had gathered out front and were screaming insults and worse at a group of police officers and Ms. Mary's husband, who they believed was trying to get rid of her. She was not insane, they insisted. Paul watched Ms. Mary get carted away. He never saw her in the neighborhood again.

Paul's first job was with the Baltimore City Welfare Department as a public assistance worker for almost a hundred families in one of Baltimore's very poor, Black communities. He saw terrible poverty and the stresses of the people coping with it. He would make home visits and notice that people were fearful when he came to their door. The job gave him his first solid multiracial group of friends. But he soon realized their crew couldn't have much of a social life. He couldn't find a restaurant or coffee shop that would allow them all in. That was Baltimore at the time.

Paul's journey at Crownsville began in graduate school. He was assigned to do field work at the hospital's admissions ward and would meet with patients who were brought to Crownsville from the Baltimore City Jail. These patients told Paul the doctors who visited the jail diagnosed them simply by staring at them through the bars. Paul remembers their commitment certificates looking identical, as though every patient who had been transferred from the jail to Crownsville just so happened to have the same symptoms and behaviors.

His second field placement was at the University of Maryland's psychiatric inpatient ward for teenagers. At that time, the hospital admitted only a few Black patients. Paul was assigned to work with a teenage

Black girl who was placed into seclusion. He clashed with the other nursing staff, who were prohibiting the girl's mother from visiting her. Paul fought to get her clearance and personally escorted the mother back to see her daughter. It was the beginning of his career working with children. And the start of him asking, What is mental illness?

Paul was drawn to the work of Dr. Thomas Szasz, a psychiatrist who forcefully argued that diagnoses were distractions from the root causes of why people are unwell. Dr. Szasz strongly opposed coercive psychiatry: he believed that mental health was an alienating and pseudoscientific concept forged by an Establishment that sought to control rather than heal. Like Dr. Szasz, Paul believed that illness was a logical response to poverty and societal trauma. That approach got Paul into some trouble in his early career, causing friction between him and other social workers who would eagerly toss around diagnostic categories. Paul preferred to think of behaviors as problems in living and coping.

When he first arrived at Crownsville in 1960, Paul remembers, he saw a mass of patients sitting around the hospital's dayrooms for hours on end without any scheduled activities or planned events to partake in. Crownsville staff were easily overwhelmed and frustrated by the patients. And so seclusion rooms and restraints were often used "for the convenience of the staff" rather than for the health of a patient. He didn't want to argue about the efficacy of any of these practices—or the rough realities of the few tools available to physicians in the first half of the twentieth century—Paul was primarily concerned with the staff's tendency to overuse tools of restraint, and how often those decisions were left unquestioned.

Administrative records and photographs from the 1950s and 1960s back Paul's view. A letter dated June 23, 1952, from Kenneth B. Jones, chairman of Maryland's Mental Hygiene Board of Review, to Maryland's governor, Theodore McKeldin, expressed rhetorical outrage about the state's funding of Crownsville:

> Why is less being done relatively to relieve the distressing overcrowding at
> Crownsville than at any of the other institutions, or why is this institution

allowed a patient per capita cost of $1,085; an amount less than any of the
other hospitals; fifty per cent less than two of them?

Jones, as chair of the state asylums' governing and monitoring body,
suggested that the government treated Crownsville with discriminatory
indifference. Being left without adequate capital, and yet subject to the
same scrutiny and standards enforced by the Mental Hygiene Board of
Review's supervision, Crownsville and its patients had been set up to fail.

Paul suspected these pressures were part of the reason the hospital
seemed unwilling to stop forcing its patients to work, cook, and make
products that it could sell. He described how employees would discuss
the fact that a higher proportion of patients at Crownsville were working
than at any other hospital in Maryland, and that the hospital was so short
on funding from the state that it "could not survive without the work the
patients did." In a February 25, 1959, memo to the chairman of the Senate Finance Committee, a state employee named John Shriver offered a
breakdown of the income and acreage of the farms at each Maryland asylum. Crownsville, with 525 acres of farmland and an income of $127,000,
outproduced all of its peer institutions. Spring Grove and Springfield, the
two largest white hospitals in the state, produced only $197 and $137 per
acre respectively, while Crownsville produced $242. Despite its chronic
underfunding and smaller patient population, Crownsville was able to
extract *substantially* higher yields than its peer hospitals. Paul became an
employee only one year after this memo was published, and he remained
concerned that government deprivation had placed unique pressure on
the hospital. Industrial therapy might have been described as therapy.
But from where Paul stood, work was work, especially when the hospital
wasn't getting enough funding to survive without it. Decades after they
had been forced to build themselves an asylum, Black patients at Crownsville were still trapped in a cycle of free labor.

On the first of each month, Crownsville produced an internally circulated "Hospital Report" in which the records and events of the previous month were detailed. These reports included data on the number
of admissions, discharges, and escapes, the status of paroled patients

temporarily living in the community, therapeutic offerings, and industrial and farm production levels. The production-related reports were the most detailed, second only to the pages tracking the number of admissions, deaths, and discharges. The July 1950 report, for example, contained an Industrial Shop Report page explaining that the office had "worked a total of ten patients on repairing beds, filling bedticks, making brooms and baskets." The report listed 339 brooms, 9 baskets, 179 bedticks, 43 repaired beds, and 2 wheelchairs for a total of 572 items prepared and sent to the storeroom. The records make no mention of connecting patients to new vocations, but they do highlight that the patients' products were stockpiled in the hospital for employee use.

A 1958 hospital report titled "Ten Year Plan and History of Crownsville" outlined the industrial objectives of Crownsville. The report explained that Occupational Therapy, Recreational Therapy, Industrial Therapy, and Music Therapy were the main components of treatment. The goal, particularly for chronically ill patients, was to achieve enough recovery to move them from music and occupational efforts and toward industrial therapy, which was described as "the rehabilitation method of choice for patients." Other therapy and recreational opportunities were reportedly organized around work duties and "scheduled at times of the day when patients [were] not busy elsewhere," when the reality is that patients had their time freed up to make space for work shifts. According to Paul Lurz, it was not uncommon for patients to have their privileges to relax outside or participate in group activities taken away if they refused to work. Although industrial therapy was a popular component of state hospital therapeutics in the 1950s and 1960s, records show that Crownsville's labor was uniquely focused on contributions to internal functions and also potentially detrimental to patient treatment and recreation. This, combined with the reliance on seclusion, created a disastrous effect on patient experiences at Crownsville.

When Howard Norton's series on "Maryland's Shame" debuted, the entire state reacted in disgust. The governor received several hundred letters and telegrams that ranged from outrage to profound sadness. Residents wrote to the paper and demanded that the legislature take action.

Just one week after the series came out, lawmakers formed a special joint committee to investigate all of the state's mental institutions. By February of the same year, then-governor William Preston Lane announced a $20 million capital improvement plan for the state hospitals, with space at Crownsville doubled.

The plan was that, over the course of several years, this investment would expand the square footage available per patient and alleviate overcrowding. The article outlined the comparative bed, recreation, and therapy space in each state hospital, noting the number of square feet currently provided and proposed for the future. In 1949, Crownsville had bed space comparable to that of the white institutions (approximately 42 square feet per patient), but it had only 1.5 square feet of therapy space per patient, whereas its peer hospitals had on average 6.3.

The planned expansions did little to remedy this. While all of the hospitals across the state were going to be expanded to an average of 60 square feet of bed space and 50 square feet of dayroom space per patient, Crownsville was set to receive about half the standard additional therapeutic space. The white institutions were to be expanded to between 10 and 11.5 square feet of therapy space, Crownsville to only 6.5. The imbalance was impossible to ignore. The government's exclusion of Crownsville from what it otherwise presented as the standard of care suggested that, at best, the development of Crownsville's therapeutic capacities was less of a priority. The state did, however, invest in Crownsville's dayrooms and sleeping spaces.

In the archives, I found a document from the early 1960s in which hospital administrators reflected on the hospital's earlier attempts at improvement and wrote, with surprising honesty, about the impact segregation and diminished social capital had had at Crownsville during the 1950s.

The administration drew a direct connection between the low status of the Black hospital and the inability to improve its programs and facilities. In the 1950s, the hospital reportedly spent $13 million on capital improvements that were solely devoted to custodial additions and increased bed space as opposed to departmental hires or therapeutics.

Despite millions of dollars spent on the hospital's infrastructure, administration acknowledged that overcrowding had only decreased by seven beds after renovations in the 1950s. The hospital leaders theorized that the expenditures were misguided, though predictable, given the low priority and position of the hospital. Haphazard expansions and an emphasis on custodial, rather than curative, spaces, they explained, were directly linked to the public's opinion of Black patients "in present day culture."

As Crownsville suffered on the inside, forces conspired against it from the outside. The white community surrounding Crownsville was becoming increasingly wary of what it perceived to be dangerous Black people roaming uncontrolled behind the hospital's walls. Crownsville became increasingly isolated, and its isolation took on many forms. At its most literal, it was "cage" seclusion cells and labor that provided neither social contact nor vocational opportunity. At its most structural, it was part of a statewide effort to maintain separation of the races at any cost.

PART TWO

Fear and Fury

1940–1960

1940: **1,438 Patients**
1960: **2,038 Patients**

CHAPTER 6

Cousin Maynard

T HE ONLY THING I EVER KNEW ABOUT MY FATHER'S COUSIN MAY-
nard was how he died. I first heard the story when I was eleven
years old.

Some of my cousins had just come to our home to visit, and as my
dad stood over the kitchen counter one night reading the paper, I inched
over to him and asked why he never talked about his cousins. In some
cases, they had lost touch or moved far away. Another cousin who had
been his close companion as a kid had been in and out of jail as an adult.
The man I called Uncle Kendal was actually a cousin, and, well, his big
brother, Maynard, was dead. I asked how, and my dad explained it to
me matter-of-factly. A cop killed Maynard. Nobody in the family had
witnessed his cousin's final moments, so everything we knew about
Maynard's killing came from the Mobile, Alabama, police department.
Everything I was going to know about Maynard came from the white
police officer who shot him within seconds of finding him.

My father is a funny combination of honest and reserved. Honest, in
that he will answer any question you ask truthfully. Reserved, in that
if you fail to ask excellent follow-ups, he will keep all the key details to
himself. At eleven, you don't ask great follow-up questions, so my dad
was able to stay at the story's surface and sidestep most of its pain. Almost
two decades later, after years of observing my own family, I've grown

convinced that when you swallow your pain it never does digest. I suspect that untreated pain curdles your blood and changes your code. It sinks into your bones, it blisters to the surface, and then it presents like diabetes, alcoholism, depression, obsessive compulsion, cancer. At least, that's what it looks like in my family. My father's and his father's pain likely have become my own unease and obsession. In changing his own DNA, he changed mine. He may remember Maynard as a cousin and friend, but his refusal to remember out loud means that, for years, I've been haunted by a dead man.

When my loved one began to struggle and I became desperate for answers, I learned to ask better follow-up questions. I started to value the time, good and bad, that people spent living, and to focus less on their worst moments. I decided to start by resurrecting Maynard.

In the summer of 1971, Maynard traded the humid and sticky city of Mobile, Alabama, for the fraught and also sticky city of Detroit. He brought all his bags, walked up two flights of narrow winding stairs, and crashed into the green-painted guest bedroom in my grandparents' house on Oakman Boulevard. There was no A/C, but two industrial fans ran up in that room around the clock to keep its guests from passing out. Maynard was about five feet, seven inches, had a short Afro, beautiful dark brown skin, and piercing, somewhat wild eyes. There was a certain confidence within Maynard; he seemed liberated and sure of himself. My dad remembers watching his older, cooler cousin get up every day, put on stylish suits, and go off in Detroit to do his own thing. During the day he would clerk for my grandfather, a local civil rights lawyer. At night, when he was around and willing to give my dad and his identical twin, Kevin, some attention, music and politics brought them together. My dad describes Maynard's taste as "far out." He talked about revolutionary, fearless stuff. The music he played made no apologies. The tracks were like nothing my father, Keith, or Kevin had ever heard in their adolescence. Maynard taught them new expletives, too, though Dad declined to tell me which ones. He pulled Keith and Kevin into his world when they were just eleven—laughing and playing music with their big cousin at the same age I was when I learned that Maynard was dead.

Maynard introduced them to the forefathers of hip-hop, blasting the Last Poets from that hot guest room. My dad remembers hearing these lyrics for the first time:

> *Guns and rifles will be taking the place of poems and essays*
> *Black cultural centers will be forts supplying the*
> *revolutionaries with food and arms*
> *When the revolution comes*
>
> *When the revolution comes*
> *White death will froth the walls of museums and churches*
> *breaking the lie that enslaved our mothers*

During dinner, Maynard could barely keep still. He'd get a little drunk and walk around the dining table, laughing and arguing with my grandparents and my dad's oldest brother, Kenny, about civil rights, Richard Nixon, and philosophy. Keith and Kevin would listen and stare. Though he was short, Maynard had a commanding and athletic presence. He carried around his own autographed copy of *The Autobiography of Malcolm X* until he passed it down to his younger brother Kendal. He would tell anyone who listened all about the latest books he had read or his theories of the world order. He liked to say that the best sport to play as a Black man was lacrosse. Why, you ask? Because it was one of the few ways you could hit a white boy upside the head with sticks and nobody could do anything about it.

Underneath the surface, an illness had been long in the making. Throughout the sixties and early seventies, Maynard had grown more fearful, morbid, and conspiratorial; he was sleeping less and less. The problem was, so were many Black people at the time. Martin Luther King Jr. had been assassinated three years earlier. The city of Detroit had burned in the long, hot summer of 1967. Police were targeting men like

Cousin Maynard here and back in his hometown of Mobile. Fear was nothing out of the ordinary.

Maynard had grown up and gone to school in Mobile right across the street from Herndon Avenue, where a nineteen-year-old named Michael Donald would hang from a tree branch ten years later. In March 1981, after a racially mixed jury failed to find a local Black man guilty of the murder of a white man, a group of Ku Klux Klan members set out driving around the city, looking for any random Black person to murder. They spotted young Michael walking back home, carrying a pack of cigarettes he had picked up for his sister. The KKK kidnapped him, beat him with a tree limb, slit his throat three times, and left his body hanging. Maynard and Kendal knew this tree. They knew its shape, its knots and wrinkles. Maynard used to drive past the tree on Herndon Avenue all the time. One of the perpetrators became the only KKK member executed for the murder of a Black person during the entire twentieth century.

In 1966 Maynard entered the University of Alabama as a freshman, a little more than two years after George Wallace, a notorious racist and the governor of Alabama, had stood in the schoolhouse door of Foster Auditorium. Wallace put on an exaggerated performance of "states' rights" in the face of federal agents as he blocked two young Black students, Vivian Malone and James Hood, from entering to register at the university and pay their semester fees. Our family had begged and pleaded: *Please, Maynard, pick any other school.* They and other Black families had heard that the Ku Klux Klan had been swarming and closely watching the college campus. As expected, Maynard went anyway, excited to stick a big, Black middle finger to any white person who made him feel unwelcome. But by the end of his first year, he started confiding in his little brother Kendal that he suspected he didn't have long to live. Kendal was terrified. The family started to wonder if something was wrong, but nobody had the words to name it, and certainly none of the tools to fix it.

Kendal, now a physician in Mobile, recalls that as Maynard made his way through college and then law school, he was often rambling about

The Man. "The Man is out to get me," he'd say. "The Man is watching me. I can't sleep," and "The Man doesn't want me to pass my exam." Kendal, eleven years his junior, would just listen quietly and try to understand. "The Man was real in the 1970s for a Black man from the South. But how do you deal with The Man?" Kendal once asked me earnestly. I fell silent. "People were out to get him, and eventually people got him. It is hard to identify or diagnose mental illness in those conditions. It makes the symptoms look logical." To my young father, though, Maynard seemed like he was more alive, like he existed somewhere closer to the truth than anyone else they really knew.

It was five years after their boisterous six months together in Detroit that a cop killed Maynard. My dad can repeat all of the facts of the shooting that occurred on October 27, 1976. But he struggles to conjure any images that are his own. He can see headlines. He remembers there were phone calls. He can't reconcile the Maynard that died on the steps of the federal building in Mobile with the Maynard who made him feel important, subversive, and free. He's not even sure if he attended the funeral. His memory went blank.

Maynard was twenty-seven, freshly graduated from Texas Southern Law School, and had been struggling to pass the bar exam. Everyone knew Maynard was hurting, but he was hiding the full extent of his paranoia. He was also keeping a terrible secret: Maynard was hearing voices.

It's estimated that a majority of people living with schizophrenia have these auditory hallucinations at some stage. They often grow stronger, more argumentative in dialogue, and become harder to ignore over time. The sounds can come as a whisper in your ear, a distant command from across the street, or a scream so loud you cannot bear it. My loved one did not hear voices, but they did report some memories of incidents, usually incredibly violent, that have not happened. Both Maynard and my loved one became trapped in loops, unable to stop verbally repeating or redescribing their fears, frustrated that people around them didn't appear to be acting with as much urgency. The illness was all-consuming, they could not pay much attention to almost anything beyond what the illness showed or told them.

According to the authorities, around 6:30 p.m. on that evening in October, Maynard drove himself to the old Federal Building at 113 St. Joseph Street. He jumped out of the car, visibly desperate, and told the first security guard that he saw, "I don't care who it is, but someone has got to take me out of the country tonight!"

The guard barricaded himself indoors. Moments later, Mobile Police Department's Officer Benny Twiggs arrived on the scene. Maynard raised a .38-caliber revolver and either lunged or ran at Twiggs. No one really knows what Maynard did with the gun, except the officer who shot him. Twiggs fired once, striking him in the abdomen. My dad's cousin died three hours later in the hospital.

Kendal received the phone call at 7:30 p.m. He remembers feeling as though the night was engulfed in an impenetrable darkness; the brightest lights on his car weren't enough, and he was convinced he might crash at any moment as he sped to the hospital. By 10 p.m., his big brother was gone.

In some ways, Kendal and, to a lesser extent, my father have been lost in a dark fog ever since. It was a death so hurtful and so strange it's made it impossible for anyone to talk about Maynard's life. Maynard, once a force of light and a loud, belligerent voice, started to retreat into a footnote of our family history. A person so ahead of their time, reduced to their last horrible seconds on earth.

Today, Kendal says he sees his brother's death as racially motivated, unnecessary, unjust. When blue lights come up behind him, he still feels his heart rate go up. He wishes there had been a framework for de-escalation or a rallying cry like Black Lives Matter—that it had been easier to find a community of people to grieve with. Instead, his brother Maynard's legacy has been summed up in headlines like "Gun-Wielding Man Shot Down by Officer." My father agrees with him. "Maybe the officer would have been slower about it, or worked harder at a peaceful resolution, if Maynard had been white," he told me. "I suspect this may have been the case." At the same time, Kendal doesn't put all the blame on Officer Twiggs or the Mobile police force. Some of my family members are convinced that death was what

Maynard wanted; that this was suicide. They didn't know what he was going through, but they sensed he couldn't take it anymore. And no Black man as conscious and culturally critical as him, they reason, would pull a revolver on a white police officer in Alabama without the full knowledge of how that encounter would end. Maynard may have been sick, but he had always, always been brilliant.

For a brief time, Kendal's father, Maynard Vivian Foster Sr., contemplated suing the Mobile Police Department. Kendal remembers looking at his dad and realizing that he was worn and weary. Maynard Sr. had finished a multi-year public battle, *Foster v. Mobile County Hospital Board*. He sued the Mobile County General Hospital, arguing that their policies had effectively discriminated against Black doctors, and, ultimately, he won. Publicly he was proud; privately, the big win had exacted a price.

December 27, 1977, exactly one year and two months after the death of his son, Dr. Maynard Foster Sr. died, too. He had beaten all the odds: graduating from a Black medical school in the mid-1900s, serving in World War II, winning a landmark case, transforming his field. Losing his first son and namesake was shattering. "It hurt too bad when Maynard died," Kendal explained. "He couldn't figure fighting it out again."

When my dad first told me so matter-of-factly that he had lost his big cousin and then his uncle, I felt so much sorrow for my daddy and for my grandparents and for Kendal. I wanted to be my dad's friend, to tell him I was sorry that he had lost a cousin who had introduced him to new ways of looking at the world. Later, I was enraged. I was angry that no one could get Maynard any help. Angry that nobody talked about Maynard anymore. Angry that young Black people like Maynard have navigated this country with the knowledge that they could be blocked from a door, hung from a tree, or shot on the steps of a federal building, so easily and violently and with impunity. That, in fact, they could *bet* on it. They could lunge toward that fate. As I got older, questions kept nagging at me. Was there a connection between the two: between living with the weight of that reality—striving to become somebody and to live defiantly in spite of it—and suffering mental trauma? Was Maynard really plagued by delusions, or was he refusing to keep quiet about the same pain and terrors that so many of our family members try to swallow whole? Were we all actually looking at the same set of facts about our existence and coming to very different conclusions about how to cope?

I asked Kendal how he's found healing, how one finds their way out of the dark fog when tragedy and illness strike. He isn't sure. "It still hurts the same way after all the years," he told me. "But talking to you is helping me. It feels good to revisit. Isn't that what you want? I don't want it to not hurt anymore. It means I've forgotten something."

CHAPTER 7

Black Men Are Escaping

IN THE WINTER OF 1954, TWENTY-ONE-YEAR-OLD URIA YODER found himself outnumbered in the dining room of the C Building at Crownsville Hospital. Uria was quiet, usually choosing to keep his distance from crowds and employee cliques, but he stood out on the grounds anyway. While other hospital workers wore lab coats, nurses' uniforms, or suits, Uria always wore modest black trousers and collarless shirts.

At his side that night was only one other male employee. Staring back at them were 102 patients. Uria had a sense of what was about to happen. He had heard the stories of what went down on this ward. It was a tinderbox.

According to newspaper reports and hospital records, everyone knew that the patients living in C were consumed by rage and resentment. Over the last two years, they had demanded better conditions. When improvements never materialized, they repeatedly ripped pipes from the radiators and walls in the dayroom, breaking infrastructure and sending water cascading down into hospital rooms, destroying mattresses, decks of playing cards, books, and shoes. Sometimes they would light mattresses on fire. The staff on this ward would scramble to regain control, exhausted after working shifts with little support in a department that often had more than a dozen job vacancies. Attendants who had clocked out for the day would be called back to the hospital to help quell the chaos.

One night in 1953, some of the staff arrived to find that their colleagues had barricaded themselves in a bathroom. As they huddled inside, patients crowded at the door holding fiery newspaper rolls like they were tiki torches. They were attempting to smoke the employees out. Uria knew some of the men, and they had managed to survive that night in February 1953 by taking turns sticking their heads inside a toilet and repeatedly flushing it and gasping for fresh air.

Riots at Crownsville were not an anomaly during the 1950s. In fact, they were expected. C Building was notorious for housing "criminally insane" patients who had been deemed unfit to stand trial, but administration, at times, crammed children and other patients into the ward's toxic mix. The building was also teeming with restless patients due to the impact of World War II. Black families had flocked from rural parts of the South to Baltimore in search of wartime jobs with the Fisher Body plant and Bethlehem Steel in Baltimore County. And with them came a new population of patients in need of support that Crownsville was, frankly, unequipped to provide.

The staff were exasperated, too. Some had been forced to accept pay cuts dating back to the Depression, and many had weathered some of the hospital's worst days during the war. At one point in 1945, ten attendants and two physicians had managed 1,700 patients alone. During another period, they had gone without access to soap or scrubbing powder for twelve terrible weeks.

The same year, *Sun* reporter Weldon Wallace wrote that the hospital's most chronically ill patients were being housed in something like a "dungeon." The area had constant issues with water pressure. Twice a day staff would bring by a bucket of water and two cups, and the patients would be forced to share the containers to get a drink. Hot water was rare, and "inmates" could not shower every day. Some patients had their own beds. Others slept on straw ticks and wooden benches. There were three toilets, three washbasins, and one tub to be shared by over ninety floormates.

Staff were openly groaning about how they wished they were working at one of the white hospitals. The turnover was frequent. But Uria wasn't one of those people. He liked working with his patients. The only time he felt nervous was at night while working the 11 p.m. to 7 a.m. shift. It could be frightening making his rounds on the ward "with lights out and having 102 men in the same room to sleep," he once wrote to me.

Patients would write to the *Afro* newspaper, begging Black journalists to investigate their housing conditions. They were aware that their disability and diagnoses had been used to discredit them, and they would plead for someone to listen. Month after month passed, and inadequate medical care, poor living conditions and health standards, and the increasing number of deceased contributed to a dehumanizing environment. A constant reminder of how society saw them and how desperate their conditions were. One night, a patient invited Uria to take a look at something he had constructed for self-defense. The patient had taken a warped piece of shoe support and sharpened it on the concrete floor like a knife. He took strips of a bedsheet and wrapped them around the other end like a handle.

When riots inevitably broke out, hours would go by before help arrived. Dozens of squad cars of armed police from surrounding counties would eventually descend upon the hospital. Tear gas and fire extinguishers would follow. Reporters would swarm around the bruised and battered attendants—but rarely did they get the chance to speak directly to the patients. A group of male "inmates" would then be identified as escapees or riot ringleaders, their names would go out in the papers, and they would eventually be carted off to Anne Arundel's county jail.

So Uria knew what came next.

Lunch trays soared through the air, chairs went flying overhead. Uria noticed some of the patients were hiding. A group of men escaped from their cells on the fourth floor. One of them took a sharpened spoon handle and stabbed the gate man on duty in the back. The guard, desperate to survive, didn't put up a fight. He stepped back, letting them rush through the ward doors and down the steps, as Uria remembers it, in an attempt to "save the attendants' necks."

Out of nowhere, a patient slammed the leg of an oak chair outfitted with metal braces down on Uria's head. Uria lifted his hands in front of his face for protection, but the patient overwhelmed him. Blood spattered from gashes the bludgeon created in his forehead and hands. He was almost knocked out.

A group of patients backed Uria and the second attendant down a hallway outside the dining room. They snatched his colleague's set of keys and let Uria and the other man escape. The two ran into an open bedroom, where they waited. And waited.

They could hear glass breaking on the floor above—patients had smashed their way into the medicine room and were grabbing what they could. Later, Uria realized he had heard patients throw his own supervisor down the second-floor stairwell. He sat still in the bedroom until he heard the sound of a police whistle. Someone came to carry him out.

For two days, Uria stayed in the hospital's nursing area, where his wrist was examined, and a doctor sewed the skin on four of his fingers and his forehead back together. Upon his release, Uria went back home to his family's rural community in Southern Maryland—a quiet and remote place where he could recover for a full month.

Uria Yoder was a pacifist. In fact, he had come to Crownsville precisely because he had been raised Amish, in a tight-knit community that fiercely opposed war and refused participation in the U.S. military's ongoing draft.

Prior to World War II, representatives of the traditional "Peace Churches," including the Quakers, Amish, Mennonites, and Church of the Brethren, held a meeting in Washington, D.C., and worked out a deal with lawmakers. The agreement was that their members would not be drafted into the army, and in exchange, they would be assigned to various programs and forms of civil service. Uria's assignment was Crownsville. The hospital offered him forty-five dollars per week to live in employee housing and work in the most intense, overcrowded, and deprived section of the hospital.

So for three years, an Amish man found himself suiting up every day to work inside an asylum. Uria treated it as a duty, carrying with him the knowledge that his Amish community may be wary of him for spending time in the "outside world."

The core issue behind Crownsville's dysfunction, and what truly set it up for violence and struggle, was the persistent funding and reputational disparity. Uria was a victim of physical violence, but he was also a victim of the bizarre and negative cultural capital associated with the state's only Black asylum. The biases that kept officials from properly funding the hospital did not just hurt the patients—they also imperiled employees.

A few years later, in 1960, the Mental Hygiene Board of Review returned to inspect Crownsville and found persistent low morale. Crownsville superintendent Dr. Charles Ward asked the board to brainstorm solutions to the "amount of prejudice which the hospital as a whole experiences." He told state leaders that this persistent prejudice had led the resident medical staff to desire work "with some white patients since the cultural and social problems of the two races differ." The staff felt not only that the institution was second-rate but that Black patients were keeping them from receiving the standard training experience. For staff, patient types and experiences were a form of capital that allowed them to advance their careers. Exclusive contact with Black patients, in other words, meant inferior knowledge and a less transferable skill set.

Dr. Ward worried that the addition of more "colored" employees would cause white applicants to stop seeking jobs at Crownsville, unless their team took action. The board said that they would hire the most competent people, regardless of race, but offered to look into the possibility of a solution. They proposed bringing in approximately one hundred white patients to Crownsville so that the professional staff could "have the training experience which they would like."

The suggestion that the presence of white patients, as a fraction of the total patient population, would increase the asylum's status and help the administration retain employees, showed how at the highest levels, the hospital could see how racism threatened its therapeutic and professional standing.

On September 17, 1955, Uria finished out his service at Crownsville and made it back to his family safely. They continue to run a produce stand in Charlotte Hall, Maryland. Every few months, he writes back and forth with his friend and former colleague Paul Lurz.

Peddling Panic

By the middle of the century, the population of Anne Arundel County was exploding. The dirt country roads and unsettling quiet that had defined the hospital's landscape in the early 1900s were starting to fill in with new construction and growing middle-class neighborhoods. The county's census had counted less than 40,000 people at the time of the hospital's founding. By 1950, there were 117,392 residents. By the 1960s, the population had almost doubled again.

As the population swelled, so did the community's awareness and concern about the asylum. Local newspaper articles reflect a population increasingly in fear of what it perceived to be hyperaggressive, hardened Black criminals living within the asylum walls.

In the 1950s and 1960s, just like the rest of the United States, people in Maryland were engrossed in cultural debates about the mentally ill. It was a time when new medications for mental illnesses were being introduced to psychiatric hospitals, raising hopes for the recovery of patients and reunion with their families and communities. Articles in *Time* magazine, *Woman's Home Companion*, and local newspapers heralded the arrival of the psychotropic drugs to American hospitals. This cultural preoccupation with mental health was reflected in popular media and literature, too. The 1960 film *Psycho*, directed by Alfred Hitchcock, sensationalized the topic of the criminally insane, as did the 1967 adaptation of Truman Capote's *In Cold Blood*. In his 1962 novel *One Flew over the Cuckoo's Nest*, Ken Kesey criticized coercive mental institutions and portrayed patients as relatable and even admirable. However, despite the widespread discussions about mental health, medicine, and therapy in many communities, Anne Arundel County and its neighboring areas had a strained relationship with Crownsville Hospital.

Some of the headlines and local commentary that came out of this period were highly racialized. As worries took on a life of their own, the media exacerbated existing divides and amplified narratives that pitted local white families against Crownsville's patient population.

The leaders of newsrooms make choices about what they cover and how often they cover it, and sometimes they can overemphasize one community's dysfunction as they downplay another's. During this period, many Black families in Maryland believed that mainstream, majority-white newspapers like the *Baltimore Sun* made selective decisions to emphasize crime, dysfunction, and negativity in communities of color in the state. With their concerns taken into account, newspapers provide a useful window into the presence Crownsville held in Maryland's cultural and social consciousness, and into the structural assumptions and prejudices at play.

The people of Anne Arundel County had great anxiety about the patients at Crownsville, and were eager to fortify, not relax, the hospital's harsh, prisonlike conditions. Often, the media emphasized stories of escapes and riots at Crownsville, and subtle differences in word choice suggested that while residents may have expected the institution to *manage* aggressive Black patients, they anticipated the *rehabilitation* of white patients.

By the late 1940s, stories about violent escapes, aggressive Black men, and the anxieties of white residents were becoming routine. The press started advancing a narrative: Black patients at Crownsville, often painted as uniquely violent and disgusting, were to remain under increased supervision. Even as white patients deserved sympathy and the benefits of rehabilitation.

In an August 1948 article published by the *Baltimore Sun* and titled "Crownsville Issue Left to Hospital Head," early community fears and a desire to expand confinement rather than reduce it were on display. The article reported that residents living near the institution had complained about the frequency of escapes and demanded the construction of a twelve-foot-high fence with guarded gates around the hospital, effectively preventing patients from venturing beyond the boundaries of Crownsville's property. White residents were advocating for the creation of a literal wall to keep Black patients at a distance.

The hospital's superintendent, Dr. Jacob Morgenstern, tried to stress the importance of outdoor therapeutic time for patients, and how a large fence or wall might interfere with their ability to treat and cure patients. The hospital's long-term goal was to hire enough employees and reduce the number of patients living together on the wards. Their aim was to separate the criminally insane patients, who required the most supervision, from the rest of the population so that the staff could better oversee patients.

The state's commissioner of mental hygiene, Dr. George Preston, responded to the growing public outrage over Crownsville's patients by proposing a system of badges and labels for patients deemed "safe" enough to have limited freedom within the grounds and nearby shops. While Dr. Preston acknowledged the valid concerns of the locals regarding the criminally insane at Crownsville, he urged citizens, in a published letter to the governor, to consider the escapes from Crownsville in a broader context.

In June, two patients escaped from the adult section of Crownsville, but both were eventually apprehended. In July, four patients escaped, with two still on the loose. Additionally, twelve patients from the division for "feebleminded" children escaped from Crownsville, with ten being returned. However, during the same period, sixteen patients left Springfield State Hospital and seventeen left Spring Grove "without permission," he explained.

The commissioner's statement was shrewdly political. He gently pushed back by informing people that the number of escapes from Crownsville was comparable to those from local white hospitals, and the majority of patients had been found and brought back. Yet, through subtle language choices, he portrayed Crownsville patients differently from those at Springfield or Spring Grove. He referred to Crownsville patients' actions as an "escape," while describing the white patients as simply "leaving without permission." The term "escape" carries a connotation of misconduct, while "leaving" implies a more casual departure. In just a few sentences, the commissioner managed to present conflicting messages, both refuting and pandering to the fears harbored by some community members regarding Crownsville patients. Through the use of descriptive cues, he subtly aligned with the concerns of the townspeople and attributed a more antagonistic intent to the patients at Crownsville than the white patients at Springfield and Spring Grove.

Four years later, the Mental Hygiene Board of Review published an "Interim Report" on the status of the criminally insane across the state. The board discussed the fact that the press was constantly writing negatively about escapes but that, in recent years, negative media attention was "largely devoted to the Crownsville State Hospital." In their report, the board members recognized that this media coverage reflected community attitudes to some extent. However, they felt compelled to highlight that the actual number of escapes by patients with criminal records was much lower than the newspapers claimed. Whether through petitions for an enormous fence or pressure on the administration to distribute badges to separate the "safe" from the unsafe, the townspeople around Crownsville had managed to reinforce differences between themselves and the patients at Crownsville. And people at the top of public health leadership were aware of it.

The fears insinuated in articles in the late 1940s became more explicit in the 1950s, with press conversations about allegedly hyper-masculine, sexually aggressive Black male "inmates" in Crownsville. Again, they reveal a community that was focused on the incarceration, and not convalescence, of the patients.

The *Baltimore Sun* article "Crownsville Residents to Ask McKeldin to Move Criminals," published in 1951, portrayed the violent escape and rap sheet of a Black nineteen-year-old named Andrew Peterson, who had been living on the criminally insane ward after a rape conviction. Peterson had seized two guards on his ward and successfully locked them into his own cell before escaping from the hospital. Not long after, authorities apprehended him just before "he and another Negro apparently were getting ready to break into a store."

The next morning, panic ensued. Twenty neighbors planned a meeting with Governor McKeldin's office to demand that all of the criminally insane at Crownsville get transferred to another maximum-security institution. A woman named Mrs. Robert C. Adams took the lead organizing the delegation. She lived only about two miles from the hospital in a wooded area. She told the paper that while residents weren't feeling hysterical, "guns were taken into the bedrooms of many homes around here Monday night."

Adams described in detail how two elderly women alone in their homes near the hospital called their neighbors for protection, and how one young woman with two small children was alone in her home because her husband was away on duty. The story painted a vivid picture that pitted white women against a lawless Black teenager. There was no statement from Peterson or a lawyer representing him. Peterson had already been apprehended and returned to Crownsville under heavy police guard. Still, the image of a deranged Black man venturing into the domestic territory of white families was enough to get guns out on people's porches. The article confirmed the community's preconceived assumptions about patients like Peterson and the sickness they represented, and it vindicated not just his own stricter incarceration but also that of any prospective escapee. The *Baltimore Sun* did not include the context that criminally insane patients like Peterson made up only a small fraction of the thousands of people living at the hospital.

Eventually, those residents got their way. A year later, in 1952, the *Sun* published a piece, "Escapes Probed at Crownsville," about how Maryland's Department of Public Works had agreed to investigate the escapes at Crownsville on behalf of local citizens.

"Spurred by community protests," they outlined, "the State Board of Public Works made available about $15,000 for steel grills and bars and new locks." The superintendent tried, once again, to explain that the root of the hospital's troubles was in the absence of an adequate staff to oversee the patient population rather than in having too few locks and bars on windows. That the hospital had 2,300 patients—1,100 more than it had space for. But instead of spending money on therapy, employee salaries, or the reduction of overcrowding, the state spent money on new tools for imprisonment—tools that they knew weren't actually going to work.

State mental health leaders were actively discussing the fact that Crownsville was in crisis. Back in September 1951, Maryland's governor,

Theodore McKeldin, had sat down with lawmakers and residents from Anne Arundel who lived around the hospital. They were furious that patients had been escaping from Crownsville into the nearby neighborhoods, and Governor McKeldin tried to explain the state's long-term goals to alleviate hospital tensions.

Then in 1952, the Mental Hygiene Board of Review wrote a report about the various ways in which patients living in the criminally insane wards could overpower employees and try to escape. They explained:

> It is not inconceivable, that a group of patients could overpower the attendant on a ward, use the keys to unlock doors, gain access to the third-floor attendant's quarters, crawl out of a window, and slide down a drainpipe to freedom. A patient brought to the doctor's office could find opportunity to break through the entrance doors to freedom, even though these doors are locked with a special key always kept in the charge-attendant's office. Patients could also gain the entrance doors from the occupational therapy shops by a running start up the basement stairs. Still another vulnerable part is the dumbwaiter from the ward dining rooms to the basement kitchen which gives unlocked access to the back of the buildings.

They never made this play-by-play public, after realizing that it could become a prospective patients' ideal "how-to" manual. But their inaction and their inability to respond to four decades' worth of overcrowded and underfunded wards and the constant exploitation of patients set the stage for further failure.

The *Baltimore Sun*'s coverage of one white felon in 1956 stands out compared to reporting on Crownsville. The story opened like this: "A nervous and visibly shaken Orville E. Hodge was removed from his jail cell tonight..."

Hodge, formerly a powerful Republican state auditor, was described as "dapper" and ambitious, hoping one day to work for the governor. That was, until he pleaded guilty to taking part in a million-dollar check-cashing scheme and looting the state's treasury. They described how he was brought to jail in a gray silk suit and put into a cell with seven other inmates. But he didn't have to stay there for long. A Springfield psychiatrist argued that Hodge, showing signs of anxiety and shame, "was suffering from nervous strain akin to wartime 'battle fatigue.'" The doctor pushed for him to be transferred to a local hospital. County authorities approved.

At Crownsville, violence and escapes continued to absorb an immense amount of local and institutional attention. And the sad irony, of course, was that the reason Crownsville was struggling to hire enough staff and to run a safe hospital was, in large part, because the state was refusing to hire anyone who was not white. This straightforward truth seemed to go over the heads of many of its white neighbors, who wanted the hospital to spend its limited resources to fortify the hospital grounds. Meanwhile, Black Marylanders living in Anne Arundel and nearby counties were desperate for Crownsville, and many other state institutions, to desegregate. Many had tried to find jobs at the hospital for years, only to be met with disappointment. White residents' commitment to segregation and employment discrimination was directly contributing to the hospital's downfall.

This disconnect on the true cost and consequences of segregation was enough to drive Black residents mad. In March 1949, the *Baltimore Sun* editors received a letter from Howard Murphy, a Black resident of Baltimore and the chairman of the Maryland Committee for Equal Educational Opportunities. Murphy wanted to express his outrage just days after reading an op-ed in the paper that had argued that equal access to higher education for Maryland's African American residents would be a waste of money.

Murphy explained to the paper's readers that the board of regents governing the University of Maryland had already made its supportive position clear, and that all of the university's programs should be open to people of every creed and color. The only thing left to do was to allow that policy to take effect.

"Sir: It seems so elemental to me," he wrote in desperation, "that I am beginning to wonder if I am not becoming a fit subject for Crownsville."

CHAPTER 8

A Burning House

We have fought hard and long for integration, as I
believe we should have, and I know we will win, but
I have come to believe that we are integrating into a
burning house.

—Dr. Martin Luther King Jr.,
as told to Harry Belafonte

FIVE YEARS BEFORE A BLACK PERSON MANAGED TO GET THEIR FOOT
in the door as an employee at Crownsville Hospital, a reporter at
the *Afro-American* newspaper gave Dr. George Preston, commissioner of
mental hygiene for Maryland, a phone call.

In the 1940s, while every news organization provided round-the-clock
coverage of World War II, the newsroom of the *Afro-American* stood
out as one of the few teams committed to investigating the treatment of
Black servicemen and the fight against segregation. Day after day, they
released new stories delving into the consequences of racial segregation
on military operations, enrollment, and the unjust denial of promotions
to Black soldiers. They often featured excerpts from the diaries of Black
servicemen, sharing their experiences directly from the front lines.

When American troops began to establish a strategic presence across
the Caribbean, the *Afro*'s reporters sharply questioned why only white

troops seemed to secure the cushier assignments in places like Cuba, where conditions were warm and relatively safe. Meanwhile, Black soldiers were being sent to Europe. Despite enduring constant discrimination, African American servicemen, including the heroic Tuskegee Airmen, made immense contributions throughout the war. But for loved ones at home, seeing their sacrifice abroad only heightened anxiety about how little access Black Americans had to every other American institution.

So on a Tuesday afternoon in September 1943, when a reporter at the *Afro* named Mrs. Elizabeth "Bettye" Murphy Phillips managed to get the mental hygiene commissioner on the line, she did not waste a second. I got a copy of the eighty-year-old transcript of their private discussion.

"The State Employment office reports 83 vacancies at present at Crownsville," Mrs. Phillips began. She wanted to know what kinds of roles were going to open, and who would be considered for them. She informed Dr. Preston that their team was receiving numerous letters from readers. "Anything that you may want to say 'off the record,' I shall respect your confidence."

"Frankly I have one interest," the commissioner replied. "That is to see that the patients at Crownsville are taken care of as best I know. Today, I am afraid of waking up some morning and finding no one who knows anything about the patients."

Mrs. Phillips wrote down a quick note to herself: the commissioner meant that he was afraid of personnel walking off the job due to "friction."

Dr. Preston continued: "Personally, I am in favor of the set-up of believing in that the colored people can take care of their own psychiatric cases. I am scared to go ahead at the moment. It would be perfectly all right if the lower-level people that we have in our employ at this time were intelligent enough to accept this situation—you know the type. You would be playing with dynamite. I think we can work the thing out if we both go along and have patience."

Mrs. Phillips pressed on. "What would be the possibility of moving the employees as a group at Crownsville?"

"It is fantastic," Dr. Preston replied, before making clear he didn't find that idea to be fantastic at all. "Mind you have 1,500 patients. No colored person in existence knows a patient by sight, knows a thing about their histories, their records, their families, their medical treatment or the management or running of the hospital. You can't just move one whole group out and another whole group in. It's too complicated. If you were dealing with a place of machinery, all right—but you're dealing with people—human beings. It's just too complicated. I believe you can work the thing out with patience."

Then, the two went off the record. As they argued back and forth awhile, Mrs. Phillips stopped typing out Dr. Preston's quotes in their entirety, instead choosing to paraphrase him. She pressed him about recent investigations into the treatment of Black patients and the leadership of Superintendent Winterode. Dr. Preston fought back, defending Winterode's "history of work and perseverance in serving the colored people." He expressed frustration with the *Afro*'s coverage of the hospital and chided the reporter. "Patience is a two-sided affair."

When their conversation went back on the record, Mrs. Phillips refused to let up.

"Now, for the record, I would like to know whether or not, how soon, or if ever, there is going to be a move made to employ colored in other capacities than cooks."

"That will come," Dr. Preston insisted. "As soon as they can demonstrate and we can find out on the basis that they can make the thing work. All I can tell you now, and I cannot tell you this for a fact, a letter has been written to the Colonel asking for a list of the vacancies that can be filled by colored people and that this is in the making."

Mrs. Phillips tried again. "Well, as this is a State Institution, don't you think he could give the colored people barred from defense industries this chance to serve?"

"At the present time, my interest is in seeing that the patients are taken care of in the best possible way! On the other hand, I am not going to set a bomb in the midst of my hospital and have it go off in my lap," he said. "You have prejudiced people also as well as we have. If we take a try and you people demonstrate it can be done, it might work, but I can't put it into the hands of people who just don't know."

As the call came to an end, Commissioner Preston added one final rub. "You have 1,500 people that have about 3,000 members of their families. I don't think you should make them any more unhappy by printing 'horror' stories. And there really isn't anything horrible about it."

A "Bomb" Is Set Off

Each day, hundreds of doctors, nurses, aides, and groundskeepers descended on the employee cafeteria for shared meals and the chance to blow off steam. In small groups, they would walk out of their wards side by side during lunch shifts and march in matching nurses' hats or bright white lab coats across the hospital's vast lawns. There across Crownsville Road stood a one-floor brick structure. Staff would gossip and smoke on the front steps, or hurry inside to secure a table for their friends.

It was 1948. And every building, every corner of the hospital, had its own difficulties and culture. The wards were severely overcrowded in the years after World War II, holding double the patients they were built to house. There had been a string of exposés in recent years, and staff had received angry letters about the all-white care teams' treatment of patients. But the lunchroom was an oasis—the one place everyone agreed was clean and great. Much of the food and dairy products were produced right there on the hospital's farm. On one side, there were grab-and-go hot dogs, hamburgers, and salads; on the other side, employees would line up, trays in hand, to wait for a variety of fresh, hot meals. Employees could go down to the dining room's basement and shoot pool and flirt. Crownsville's teams often built trust in the cafeteria—it was where friendships were made, where they played table tennis, and where secrets were shared. At least before the day Vernon Sparks arrived.

After finishing his master's degree from New York University, Vernon Sparks set foot on Crownsville's grounds for the first time in 1948. On paper, he was exceptional. He was the son of a Pullman porter and a homemaker. Vernon was an athlete, choir tenor, and veteran. After serving in World War II and being honorably discharged, Vernon returned home, deeply affected by the horrors he had seen abroad and searching for a way to continue serving people. He received multiple degrees in history and psychology.

The hospital had long struggled to attract candidates with Sparks's credentials and expertise. White doctors with his experience preferred the university systems or Springfield and Spring Grove. Crownsville was lucky to have someone with his résumé apply. At the time, according to longtime employees, several of the doctors out on the wards were physicians who had no mental health training whatsoever. The hospital desperately needed someone who knew what they were doing.

The only problem was Vernon was Black. In fact, he was the first licensed Black psychologist in the state of Maryland. There were a few Black people working as cooks in the back, and a few farmhands who worked out in the fields with patients. But there had never been a Black member of the hospital team, and never a Black person in the dining hall. The "bomb" Commissioner George Preston had imagined back in 1943 had arrived, and he was walking into Crownsville.

News of Sparks's first day spread fast. Some of the white staff began grumbling that, if this was a sign of things to come, they would soon quit. They wanted managers to know that none of them would agree to live in the hospital's employee housing if it became integrated.

Vernon's friend and future colleague Dr. Jim Ballard told me that he believed Vernon understood what he was walking into. His New Jersey accent seemed to punctuate every difference between him and his Southern colleagues, but Jim Ballard remembered his friend as radiating a sort of calm positivity. "Vernon could've integrated with a group of rocks."

Vernon also walked in that day knowing he had an advocate and protection. The new superintendent, a Jewish man named Jacob Morgenstern, had just replaced Robert Winterode. The man that Black patients and families had for so long seen as an "overseer" of sorts was gone. Morgenstern would have Vernon Sparks's back, and he told him so in no uncertain terms.

Dr. Sparks had returned from battlefields to a country that had not been particularly grateful to its servicemen of color. Surviving that job had required patience. This one would, too. His friends describe him as having entered the hospital gracefully, pretending he was unaware of the whispers around him. Dr. Ballard recalled how Vernon Sparks's approach made his colleagues—even those who had been convinced he wouldn't be a good "fit"—feel like they were the smartest in the room. He purposefully disarmed them. "He was one of those guys that always made you feel like you were in charge," Ballard told me. "You know, I'll lead you but you'll think you're leading me?"

Dr. Ballard, now eighty-four years old, sat with me and his two adult children one evening in the Belt family home, a stone's throw from Crownsville Hospital's campus. We spent hours talking about his career and his friendship with Sparks. He explained that Black professionals had to carry a constant duality—a split sense of self—at that time and, arguably, even now. Although he admired Vernon and felt close to him, the two men wouldn't let each other know too much about certain parts of themselves. They wouldn't let their *real* militant beliefs about race, class, and America slip out into the hospital setting. Some things had to go unsaid. The two of them were trying to be psychologists and believed that as Black men, they would be measured by strict professional yardsticks.

Still, their psychological practice was quietly informed by a belief that this country had never yielded Black Americans a complete and secure self-consciousness. They observed in their patients that the world seemed to always tell them that Black people were not really American—that they were not professional, not smart. They often lacked a sense of security and a sense of place. The two doctors realized it was only sheer will that could keep some of their patients from being torn apart by the messages they'd received. During group therapy with patients at Crownsville, Dr. Ballard would tell them, "The reason you're in the hospital and I am not is that you allow people to see the part of you that is nonconforming. If you came to my house at about eleven o'clock at night, and you saw me and my wife, you would say 'Well, what's the difference in what Dr. Ballard does and what I do?'" Dr. Ballard and Dr. Sparks would open up to their patients, but they kept most of the details of their personal lives from their white colleagues.

Superintendent Morgenstern could insist that white staff work alongside Vernon, but he couldn't shield the doctor from all of their vitriol. When a majority of the white staff refused to eat in the same room with him on his first day, without protest, Vernon walked to a separate back room to finish his meals.

He was surprised one afternoon when a white administrative assistant named Ellen Stoutenberg was in the back room waiting for him. She was sitting there with her tray, determined to make Vernon feel like he had a friend. For the first few weeks, the two planned to eat all of their meals together, quietly defying the de facto segregation enforced by their colleagues.

One afternoon, Superintendent Morgenstern walked in and put an end to it. He asked Vernon and Ellen to enter the dining room and take a seat. They agreed. The two walked in side by side and the room fell quiet. From then on, the cafeteria at Crownsville was desegregated.

The Trouble Integrating

In September 1957, Gertrude Belt was at her wit's end. She and her husband, Freddy, were working seven days a week. And yet, it seemed like there was never enough money around to feed their three little ones under the age of seven. Freddy, a self-taught builder and stone cutter, was always optimistic. He smiled even when he was a little worried or mad. But Gertrude was afraid. She went knocking on doors all over Annapolis, looking for a business that might need her help. Finally, one Monday morning, a local nursing home in the city offered her a job. Gertrude prayed that these twelve-hour shifts scrubbing floors, folding linens, and running baths for elderly white Annapolitans might help her finally get ahead. She had cycled through as a cook and cleaner for many of the families in the area. Maybe this role would lead to something secure.

The following Monday, Gertrude asked the nursing home manager about her pay. He handed her twelve one-dollar bills for a full week's worth of her labor. She'd been cheated. But it wasn't the first time. There was nobody to report it to, no union or agency.

Today, when Gertrude talks about this period in her life, she still pauses to catch her breath. She rushes through some of her words, like the memory of trying to survive is still biting at the back of her heels. She tells me this story as we relax together in the living room of her 2,000-square-foot home on Hawkins Road. She's filled the home with vintage furniture and photos of her kids, family friends, and Freddy's smile. I marvel at her late husband's intricate woodwork. He built most of the home by himself.

Something about those twelve bucks broke Gertrude's spirit that day. It might have been because exactly three years earlier, in late September 1954, Gertrude had been heavily pregnant with a fourth child. She had been tired but bursting with excitement and had already chosen a name: Linda Lee. Gertrude was working in a wealthy doctor's home at the time and couldn't afford to take time off work—not with a newborn on the way. So she worked on her feet all day, cooking meals, cleaning silverware, and running after other people's children. And then one afternoon, she felt a strange sensation in her back and between her legs.

She looked down and watched as blood spilled out onto the floors of the home she had been hired to clean. Gertrude panicked—no other adults were home. She walked slowly up the winding staircase, gripping the banister as she made her way to the second floor. She hurried to find the family's phone and rang their neighbor for an ambulance. "I was scared," she told me. "I was ashamed to make a mess of their nice home."

Bleeding out, Gertrude was rushed to Anne Arundel Medical, the premier medical center in the city. It was notorious for barring Black patients and refusing to deliver Black babies. Upon her arrival, she could hear white doctors and administrators argue over whether or not to help her. "If I send her out, she won't make it," she heard one doctor yell. She knew something bad was happening to Linda Lee, and that every minute would matter.

At that time, Black mothers typically gave birth at home or traveled to see Black doctors in Washington, D.C. Gertrude doesn't remember how much time went by, but eventually she was suddenly rushed inside for a cesarean section. She gave birth to Linda Lee and brought her fourth baby home. That fall and winter were so cold, and their shack in Sherwood Forest had no heat or proper insulation. Three months later, Linda Lee died on Christmas Day, from what doctors told Gertrude was "some kind of pneumonia." I asked her if she thought Linda Lee's stressful birth and premature death were related. Gertrude had no way of knowing.

Three years later, as Gertrude held those twelve dollars in her fist, she rode home on the bus and she cried. It was on that bus, surrounded by strangers, that years of domestic labor came to a head. She felt the families she cared for were entirely indifferent to her survival. Work had taken everything from her, including her child. As she walked home from the bus stop, a woman pulled her car over and called out to the visibly heartbroken Gertrude. She introduced herself as the director of nursing at Crownsville Hospital. She wanted to know if Mrs. Belt needed a job. She would have a contract and a salary.

The job would be tough on Gertrude; Crownsville had only recently started to hire Black people, and she had never worked with psychiatric patients before. She had cleaned many homes but had never sanitized medical equipment or been asked to place maggots and leeches on a patient to clean their lesions. Gertrude was barely five feet tall—and at Crownsville, male and female employees alike were expected to restrain unruly patients. But Gertrude was tired. She was drained from cleaning wealthy white people's homes. Her new job would give her consistent wages and a safety that was rare for Black women who were doing domestic work in those neighborhoods, who had to watch their backs while working to feed their families.

Gertrude's first few years at Crownsville allowed her and Freddy to save money for the first time. She would come home at the end of the week and stash cash into an old juice can that she had converted to a piggy bank. By 1960 they had saved $3,000, and the couple purchased a plot on the corner of Crownsville and Hawkins Roads for $1,000. A little over a year later, they moved their children from the wooden shack in the forest to a one-floor house that her husband built from the ground up. Over time, there would be a chimney, a garage, and a garden.

The hospital changed their lives financially, and it also allowed their kids to finally be in a better position. Gertrude, who had dropped out of high school when she got pregnant with her first child, was now going to send her three children to a public school in rural Anne Arundel. She had heard that theirs would be one of only two Black families in the entire school system—her kids would be among the first to integrate. All Gertrude could think about, though, was that the school's facilities were state-of-the-art and its reputation stellar. She hadn't considered the pitfalls and possible humiliations of integration.

On her daughter Faye Belt's first day at their new school, a yellow bus pulled up on the corner of Crownsville Road. A white driver opened the doors, and as Faye and her brother bounced into a first-row seat, he barked, "Get to the back." Her brother, Fred, got up immediately. Faye refused. She ran home that night and told her mom. It was the first sign that although Gertrude had brought her family into a new life, these institutions might not receive them with the same excitement. On the contrary, they could embarrass and even degrade her and her children. Looking back, Gertrude sees the risk. But life had taught her and Freddy how to fight, how to recover when you've been kicked down. Little children like Faye weren't ready to shoulder that burden.

At school, Faye was the only Black child in her class. Her teacher, a man who doused himself in cologne and never seemed to wash his hair, looked floored whenever she would read passages of their textbooks out loud. Nobody in the class believed Faye could read.

She started to think her teacher was strange. She didn't like how he made his students face a whiteboard to the front, even as he sat back at his desk in a corner far behind. She was confused when he started to ask her to come visit his desk and when he started to touch her and rub her legs. She felt sick when he started to undo her pigtail braids and finger through her tight coils. She froze when he started to put his hands beneath her clothing and into her underwear. Faye would stand there silent in the back of the room with her eyes concentrated at the whiteboard ahead, waiting for her teacher to stop.

She didn't have words for what was happening. Faye would come home looking a mess, and Gertrude would scream at her. But Faye was too ashamed to explain. Instead she tried to shrink away and out of sight. She stopped raising her hand to answer questions, hoping the teacher might forget she was there. The confident, sassy, athletic girl grew quiet. Her grades started to slip, and she didn't have the energy to do her homework. At home, she'd steal money out of her mom's purse. It got harder and harder to bottle up what was boiling inside. When her classmates made fun of her, she started to shove back. Her teacher and her classmates were no longer impressed—now Faye was an aggressor.

The Belt family had access. They had more money. Their kids were in the "good" school. And yet, Gertrude's daughter was failing. She had unknowingly placed her youngest in danger.

Within a year, she realized the mistake she had made. Before Faye had finished the fourth grade, Gertrude pulled Faye out of the school and placed her into a predominantly Black school called Parole Elementary. Her new administrators, recognizing that Faye was hurting, immediately assigned her a counselor who checked in on her and helped her manage her anger. They encouraged her to join the choir and had an instructor teach her deep breathing exercises. While Faye didn't fully process the sexual assault with a therapist until years later, she came back to life the following school year. She started reading again and felt less alone.

"I was always internally dealing with that," she explained to me. It had been too much for a small child to figure out how to respond to abuse all while being socially and racially isolated at school. At that age, Faye didn't understand what it meant to be one of the first students to integrate a school system. She had never asked to be a pioneer. At Parole, she could relax with friends she knew from the neighborhood and be a *kid* for just a while longer.

Soon, Crownsville Hospital would teach Gertrude painful and personal lessons about integration. Whether they liked it or not, she and many other Black employees hired throughout the late 1940s and 1950s became symbols of change and discomfort. While their jobs provided opportunities for upward mobility, they were also on the receiving end of intense resentment and hostility from white colleagues. At times, they experienced the same degrading treatment and isolation that had long been endured by the patients.

During Gertrude's early days at Crownsville, she would arrive for her shift and stand in a line outside with a dozen other women. They'd wait as their supervisor walked past each and every one of them to make sure there wasn't a single hair out of place.

The first thing Gertrude noticed about her patients in A Building was that many of them had no clothes. Sometimes they were naked, often they had only a thin hospital gown or cotton dress tied loosely from behind, exposing their backsides. For much of the day they sat on the floor because there weren't enough chairs to go around. Several of the wards were utterly chaotic—there were children sleeping among adults, two people sharing a single twin-sized bed. The new employees would whisper about wards that were like snake pits. Gertrude and the other new nurses would step onto those floors together and try to keep each other safe. They would enter with their arms and elbows linked together, walking two by two and back-to-back. The hospital was overwhelmed, and the women worried that without a buddy system, they wouldn't be able to see a patient approach or an object flying in their direction.

When the winter came in 1957, one of Gertrude's assignments was to walk across the campus with her patients three times a day for breakfast, lunch, and dinner. It seemed like there was always a thick layer of snow or frost on the ground that year. Most patients had no shoes. She noticed many of them had feet covered in blisters. Others had blotches of black and gray skin where frostbite had sunk in and killed off their blood vessels. Gertrude would escort one small group of patients over to the dining room at a time. She'd bring them in, sit them down at communal tables, and remove their shoes as they got comfortable. As they ate, she'd trudge back across the lawn to A Building and hand the shoes over to the next group of patients. Many of the patients knew how to make and sell shoes. Gertrude wondered why nobody had brought them any. In time, she and her friends started bringing in their own old clothes and accessories to hand out when they could.

Many of the white employees had come to Anne Arundel from far away, often from rural counties deeper in Dixie. In Gertrude's view, they didn't seem to understand or like the patients, and often avoided coming close to them. The previous hiring system at Crownsville had allowed white candidates to benefit from a less competitive applicant pool and process. Many had little more than a high school education. Black nurses and doctors like Sparks, on the other hand, typically competed for a handful of spots, and many of them had multiple degrees.

Every few days, Gertrude would sit her patients down on the floor between her legs. She would squeeze them between her knees as she shampooed their hair and carefully combed their curls out. When she finished, Gertrude would mop and scrub the floors by herself. It was a hospital—but her manager had not hired professional cleaning and sanitation staff. In the 1960s, her close friend Dorothea McCullers, a talented seamstress, came to work at Crownsville, too. The two women would try to find or make the best clothing they could, and Dorothea would fix tattered linens and make custom items for patients in need.

The women were often the primary breadwinners in their families. Gladys Kent, a single mom and licensed practical nurse from Calvert County, Maryland, would bring her son Milton with her on her overnight shifts. Milton Kent, now a veteran of Baltimore journalism and a professor at Morgan State University, remembers going to sleep in borrowed hospital beds until his mom finished up her rounds at seven in the morning. He would listen to patients moan and cry, and try not to let the sounds that echoed off the sterile tile floors wake him from his sleep. Mostly, he just remembers deep gratitude for his mom finding a way to take care of him and his siblings. "She made a thirty-minute drive each way, five times a week, late at night as a Black woman driving alone," Milton told me.

When Gertrude first arrived at Crownsville, a Georgia-born doctor named Charles Ward had recently become the new superintendent. He loved to garden and make improvements to Crownsville's property, and he'd walk around and strike up casual conversations with the staff. When snowstorms came, he would get out on a tractor and clear roads by himself or deliver food to the dorms on foot. It caught some of the Black nurses off guard in a good way. They felt like he cared about them and wanted the patients to live somewhere beautiful.

At times, though, they were troubled by his behavior around campus. Several nurses recalled seeing Dr. Ward high on what they suspected was meth. He'd drive recklessly around the campus in a sports car, or he'd show up looking like he hadn't slept in days. When he was fired a few years later, for allegedly driving on a revoked license, overusing amphetamines, and using bad checks, he refused to vacate the hospital premises. Black staffers protested the firing and wrote letters on his behalf. They tried not to judge his substance abuse. It mattered to them that he was kind.

He wasn't the only one using drugs, either. Some of the white nurses and aides used drugs on the job, even as they worked with patients who had, in some cases, been forced into Crownsville for drug or alcohol use. A few of the white aides could not read or write, and would ask their Black colleagues to complete patient reports for them. It frustrated some of the new Black employees, who felt that they didn't have the luxury of making mistakes or relying on others.

Incompetence and overt hostility from white staff were often met with restraint from the small but growing clique of Black employees.

One of the hospital's first Black nurses told me that once, during her first few weeks of work, she walked out of Crownsville's campus to pick up food at a local café. When she arrived at the sandwich shop, she overheard a conversation between white colleagues. One of them was seated at a table inside with her back turned, telling a friend that she wished Crownsville could've stayed the way it was. The Black nurse took a deep, weary breath and turned around. She knew better than to confront them or fight. She walked back to the hospital.

Sarah Maddox, an aide and nurse who started at Crownsville in 1952, experienced a rough adjustment period. She became a licensed practical nurse (LPN), and she worked across the grounds serving a variety of patients, from those with epilepsy (who were routinely institutionalized throughout the twentieth century) to children with developmental disabilities. "A lot of these people [white staff] were not qualified; they wore nursing caps but they were not nurses," she once said in an interview with social worker and historian Vanessa Jackson.

One afternoon, in her cap and an ironed nurse's dress, Sarah made her rounds on the infirmary and heard a Black female patient ask for a nurse. She walked over to their bed and said confidently, "I'm a nurse." The woman shouted back, "I want a real nurse. Don't you dare put your Black hands on me!"

She realized that even Black patients had internalized and reinforced the racial hierarchy at Crownsville and saw Sarah, as the only Black woman on the ward, as a signifier of inferior care. Sarah had to come to terms with the fact that she was working with hostile white colleagues, but also with people who had never imagined someone who looked like them would be allowed to walk through Crownsville's doors as anything other than a patient.

Black nurses learned to listen intently to what their patients had to say. Sometimes the patients would tell staff they had arrived at Crownsville after stealing small items like fruit or candy. Police officers in Annapolis had picked them up and dropped them off in the admissions wing. They had committed crimes of poverty but didn't have a technical mental health diagnosis. Years of living in confinement and being treated like an outcast, however, would eventually make anyone appear sick. "They just picked up the habits of the people that were there," one nurse told me. "And therefore, they were labeled mentally ill."

Other patients were fearful and quiet when the staff came around. They had been called racial slurs and seen horrors some of the new employees could not imagine. "But when you are used to being called different kinds of names," one nurse said, "you fear the people who are actually there to take care of you." White staff and local residents alike seemed to view the hospital as a dumping ground. Betty Hawkins, a former nursing director, recalled witnessing one white family stop by Crownsville and ask to leave an elderly family member at the hospital for a week while they went on vacation. She felt pressure to be at work at all times and often accepted overtime shifts. She worried about what would happen to patients when she wasn't around.

One afternoon, a Crownsville nurse took a group of patients out for a field trip to Carr's Beach, the beach designated for Black families just south of Annapolis, and noticed a man named Joe Lee talking to her patients. He didn't seem to mind that they were different, and was patiently demonstrating the different strokes and showing them how to swim.

The nurse walked up and asked him why he would do that. "Just because they're a little different doesn't mean they don't deserve to swim and play," Joe said, according to his daughter Barbara. Crownsville hired Joe as the head of recreation in 1957.

Joe Lee's goal was to get patients up and moving. He took them bowling and organized baseball games and hospital talent shows. Joe recruited his mom, Lillian, to experiment with hosting music therapy and dance therapy at the facility. Soon enough, staff from other hospitals were coming by to take notes. Joe managed to get the administration to build a space dedicated to recreation and named it after the Black and Italian-American baseball star Roy Campanella. In 1963, they hired his daughter Barbara's future husband, Thomas Arthur, to help out for a summer internship that turned into a full-time job.

At the time, Thomas was majoring in music. Crownsville wasn't really part of his life plan so much as it was an opportunity to make money while he was finishing his degree. But with each new patient he met, Thomas became more invested. He couldn't stop questioning why some of these people had been admitted to the asylum in the first place. He started brainstorming how he could create opportunities for them to get away from Crownsville's grounds and to express themselves creatively. He was no Eagle Scout—he had never spent much time outdoors—but Thomas somehow convinced the hospital to let him plan camping and hiking trips in a park called Camp Puh'tok near Monkton, Maryland, in Baltimore County. He would bring twenty patients at a time to stay in cabins, and they would laugh and figure out how to make a fire and cook some food for a few days.

When they returned from the trips, Thomas made it his priority to write reports for the administration, detailing the emotional and mental progress each participant had made in the outdoors. He desperately wanted them to go home. He considered it a win when, weeks or months later, he'd run into old patients at his favorite local jazz clubs.

The Arthurs became part of Gertrude's small but tight-knit group of Black friends at the hospital. When one of their friends was tired, or gearing up to work a double shift, Gertrude would tell them to head over to her house. Go crash on the couch and get some rest. They were all burning the candle at both ends, often one of only two employees on a shift assigned to hundreds of patients. Gertrude's children would come home from school and see their mom's friends knocked out in their hospital uniforms on the couch in the living room.

The patients who grew close to Gertrude started to spread the word—they all figured out where the Belt house was, too. Faye was little but she was never afraid when she found them waiting in the family's yard. Adolescent patients would ask Faye to play board games or baseball. One morning before school, the kids, Gertrude, and Freddy were eating breakfast when they heard the engine of Freddy's pickup truck rev up in the driveway. They ran outside to find a patient frantic in the front seat, doing his best to figure out how to back the truck up and get out of Dodge. Faye's parents would just chuckle at stuff like this. They'd call a friend working at the hospital and ask them to come pick the patient up. Sometimes, Faye and her siblings, who were still just kids, would walk the patients back to their rooms before any administrators knew they were missing.

The hospital's records reflect the racial tension, low morale, and growing pains at every level of the hospital's operations. In September 1957, the same month that Gertrude started her job and just a few weeks after President Dwight D. Eisenhower passed the first civil rights legislation since Reconstruction, Maryland's Mental Hygiene Board of Review visited Crownsville for a routine inspection and meeting.

In the minutes taken during the meeting, Gwendolyn Lee, a Black employee and the head of Crownsville's Social Service Department, expressed concern about "the extreme turnover and poor morale of the hospital employees." Crownsville was in crisis, as she saw it, for two reasons: the hospital was isolated from commercial centers and there was no

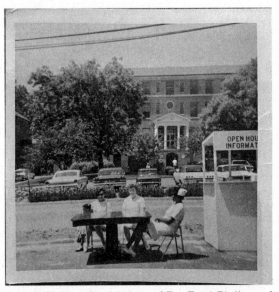

Andrea Phillip, the daughter of Dr. Errol Phillip and
Joyce Phillip, visited staff waiting at an information desk
in the late 1960s. The children of employees would explore
the hospital grounds and interact with staff and patients.
Photo courtesy of the Phillip family.

public transportation, and its status as a segregated facility was destruc-
tive. She warned leaders that staff suffered from a "low opinion of themselves and the hospital," and resources were so scarce that Crownsville's
professionals, the only doctors and nurses working with Black patients in
the state, could not travel to national and state conferences. She explained
how, since the effort to integrate, "they had had an even harder time getting well-trained workers as they go to the other mental hospitals." White
employees were fleeing Crownsville. She confirmed that 43 percent of the
staff had turned over since 1956.

Every week in the 1950s, it seemed like a new, small cluster of Black
men and women would arrive to take their place. Gertrude didn't miss
the people who left. She wanted to build a new sense of community. She
started to throw dinners and dance parties for the Black doctors and nurses
in her basement. She invited patients who were her children's age to attend
sleepovers and family dinners. Only a decade prior, the head of mental
health systems in the state had told a Black reporter that "no colored person
in existence knows a patient by sight, knows a thing about their histories,

their records, their families, their medical treatment or the management or running of the hospital." Gertrude and her friends may have been new, but they were wise. They heard white colleagues whispering about them, and caught them rolling their eyes. They sensed that state leaders like Dr. George Preston had doubted that they knew a thing about their own people and mental healthcare. But they didn't pay them much mind. They knew they were starting to make a difference.

❧

Black nurses and aides weren't entirely alone in the painstaking work of reform. Crownsville was a place of stability and community for another group of outsiders. When Dr. Jacob Morgenstern took the reins as Crownsville's superintendent in 1947, the hospital was a relic of a fading but stubborn era. From its inception, Crownsville had been a reflection of its state's policies and attitudes relating to race, criminality, labor, and healthcare. Despite its location on the North Atlantic coast, large parts of Maryland were firmly and culturally part of the Dixie South. State leadership from the governor's mansion down to the local city councils was

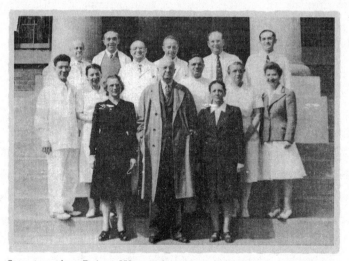

Superintendent Robert Winterode surrounded by his top doctors and administrators in 1948. Dr. Jacob Morgenstern, a Holocaust refugee wearing glasses on the far left, would soon succeed him and transform Crownsville. Photo taken by Cassandra Giraldo of records in the Maryland State Archives.

moving at a snail's pace on the question of integration. But Morgenstern was deeply uncomfortable in the antebellum hospital structure. He had to act with urgency, in no small part because he had just barely survived this kind of apartheid system himself.

In March 1938, Adolf Hitler marched his troops over the border in Germany and declared the annexation of Austria. Jacob Morgenstern, a Polish-born longtime resident of Vienna, was living there with his wife, Gisela. Gisela had converted to Judaism in 1935, as Europe was beginning to turn its back on their people. Within the first four years of their marriage, Jacob and Gisela had co-owned a pharmacy and welcomed their first child together, a daughter named Doris. The young family watched as the laws that had reshaped Germany came down upon Austria, quickly and systematically denying Jewish people their rights. That summer, Morgenstern was forced to close his medical practice and surrender his car, bank accounts, and all valuables. Then the Gestapo seized him.

Just before the Nazis planned to send Dr. Morgenstern to a concentration camp, the family received a telegram. Cousins living in New York wrote to officials, promising that they would sponsor the entire family in the United States. Jacob Morgenstern was released on one condition: leave Austria, and everything you own, immediately.

Jacob, Gisela, and Doris spent a year living in Paris with the help of one of his former patients. There the family waited for the United States to approve their visas. One month before the Nazis took France, the Morgensterns sailed to New York.

American medical facilities did not accept European licenses, forcing Morgenstern to return to school to study English and complete a medical internship on Staten Island. One day he came across a posting that read: "Immediate position for a Junior Physician at Crownsville State Hospital, Crownsville Maryland. The hospital is a psychiatric facility for Negro patients, located in a rural area equidistant from Baltimore and Washington, D.C."

He had never before practiced psychiatry. But the family's financial picture was becoming dire: they were dependent on charity from Jewish organizations, and they desperately needed resources to bring Jacob's mother and sister to safety in the United States. Crownsville represented security and opportunity. His daughter, Doris, once wrote for the Jewish Museum of Maryland, "It was a way to begin anew."

When the Morgensterns arrived on campus, there were no antipsychotic medications yet. Patients were more likely to die than find a path to recovery. Doris told me she remembers her father doing the work of multiple doctors at once, and warning that he might not make it in the job for long.

Doris was just a child at this point in her father's career, and her first memories of Crownsville are mostly of scenic farmland and intimidating brick structures. But certain experiences stuck with her. I interviewed Doris just before her eighty-third birthday, to understand the life at Crownsville that she witnessed both through her father's work as a doctor and her mother's experience after becoming a laboratory technician at the hospital. When Doris and I first spoke, I could tell she was nervous. She is proud and fiercely protective of her father's legacy. She's grown tired of the distorted, one-dimensional depictions of asylums in popular culture. Securing the interview took time and trust, but as we eased into the conversation she opened up about her father's achievements.

As a small child, Doris would stare up at hospital buildings as she walked from their house to visit her mother's lab. She would listen to loud and unfamiliar sounds that patients would make on the wards. The Morgensterns, unlike the Winterodes, tried to treat patients like extended family members. Doris remembers her parents inviting employees and patients to dine with them at home. One patient, Alma, moved out of the hospital and into her family's home for a while. Alma taught Doris how to embroider, and they would sit together and write poetry as her parents worked.

Not long after their arrival, Morgenstern discovered that his mother and sister had been denied entry to the United States. "My grandmother, his mother, had just fallen and broken her arm when they went to the U.S. Embassy," Doris told me. "She was denied because they were only taking in able-bodied people." After his failed attempt to bring his loved ones to America, her father was constantly preoccupied. "My father was the kind of person that really worries a lot. He was not really a cheerful person. And I think things weighed on him quite a bit," she explained. Morgenstern himself had barely made it out of Europe alive. He turned his attention to his patients and worked long shifts into the night.

The patients' trust in the existing staff was thin, as chronic neglect and overt racism had eroded potential therapy. Doris's parents would often go into the hospital at night to make sure that the patients were properly monitored and that the employees were behaving appropriately during their shifts. The extra work and close supervision were as much a testament to their anxieties and management styles as they were a product of the hospital's underfunding. Even as a child, Doris understood that Crownsville was struggling. She could overhear her parents talking about how there was a "skeleton staff."

In 1947, Jacob Morgenstern was appointed superintendent. Doris remembered the family being asked to move into Robert Winterode's old house, a big plantation-style estate home with many rooms. Doris remembered entering "the big house" and finding it completely barren. But before her mother, Gisela, could start to redecorate, staff made clear that her taste had been deemed too "foreign" and unsuitable. According to Doris, Gisela's new administrative assistant insisted on guiding her mom through the decoration process. It seemed as though others saw their Jewish family as needing some assistance adjusting to Southern culture.

Morgenstern spent those early years reading about psychiatry and trying to bring in new forms of psychological testing for patients. In all the chaos and injustice, he saw a profound opportunity to reform. He noticed that many of his patients were suffering from debilitating paresis, advanced paralysis, and disability from late-stage syphilis. At the time, syphilis was spreading within many poor Black communities. The disease had become heavily stigmatized, and even after the advent of penicillin, white doctors often refused to give Black people suffering with syphilis proper healthcare. Morgenstern decided to administer one of the few available therapies. He asked his staff to inject malaria-infected blood into patients to manufacture a high fever. It didn't always work, but when it did, it seemed to stop the bacterial infection.

Morgenstern was deeply uncomfortable with the divide between the staff and the patients. He could see how little the staff seemed to connect to the patients' stories, neighborhoods, and interests. Himself a refugee, he recognized this system for what it was. It reproduced racial and medical hierarchy, it shielded the white staff from discomfort and job competition, and it heaped dysfunction on vulnerable patients.

The Morgensterns allowed Winterode's staff to decorate their home, but they were not going to allow the old culture to keep ruling the hospital. Less than a year into his leadership at Crownsville, Morgenstern aligned himself with local NAACP chapters. With their support, he ignored warnings from several state leaders and made it known to them that he would fight for integration. He hired a full-time employee to oversee volunteer services and asked them to find locals willing to plan parties and offer vocational services to Crownsville's patients. Several family members of Janice Hayes-Williams, the local historian, came to the hospital to do just that. Doris recalled her father ignoring the bitter opposition, even as the hospital's neighbors told newspapers and politicians they opposed her father's reforms. They were convinced that desegregation would breed bitterness and that violence would soon follow. "Time proved them wrong," she once wrote.

It was in this environment that Morgenstern hired Vernon Sparks as a staff psychologist. And shortly thereafter, he would bring on Gwendolyn Lee as a social worker and Crownsville's supervisor of social services. Interdepartmental hiring of Black employees didn't happen overnight; strides were made through deliberate, slow effort. Gisela worked closely with her husband—her lab was one of the first sections of the hospital to desegregate. But for years, the farm and laundry departments—where patients were frequently put to work—remained controlled by entirely white staff. The social service department, where employees labored to reconnect patients with kin or find young children a home, was entirely Black from Gwendolyn Lee's appointment until the 1960s. In 1949, there were 1,800 patients and 392 staff members. Just five of those employees were Black. By 1956, there were 2,300 patients and 745 staff members, 326 of them Black.

Morgenstern managed to move thoughtfully and quietly about the hospital grounds while simultaneously creating seismic departmental shifts all around him. Slim and standing just five foot seven, he was not an imposing man. Looking back, many employees believed it was this quiet but firm style of leadership that allowed people like Jacob Morgenstern and Vernon Sparks to transform Crownsville. Both Jacob and Vernon had been forever altered by war, eugenics, and dehumanization. Both men had traveled through Europe and studied in New York. But in Maryland, their missions converged. It was an outsider and a refugee—not one of Maryland's cultural or political insiders—who were able to see Crownsville's truth and move without fear to improve it.

On January 27, 1953, friends and esteemed colleagues gathered in the cafeteria that Jacob Morgenstern had once desegregated. Everyone was huddled there to honor the contributions of the man who had changed the face of the hospital and, for the first time, put its patients first. Morgenstern had received an offer to become the new director of correctional psychiatry at the Department of Mental Hygiene. He thanked everyone there for their support and dedication, as he mourned the end of five tumultuous and transformational years. "Many of my friends are asking, 'Why?'" he said to the crowd that night. "Well, I still wonder myself…"

In a letter he sent out to the Crownsville staff, Morgenstern revealed that he had a desire to spend more time working with patients. "My administrative duties have unfortunately kept me too much away from the wards and direct contacts with patients." The fighting and negotiating had become too much. He planned to stay connected to the people and his cause. "Too much of myself has been rooted here…I intend to continue the ties with the hospital and with my friends here who have helped me to carry the burden of this immense job and have helped me to make it a good one."

Vernon Sparks would remain at Crownsville for a quarter of a century, leading a groundbreaking team that expanded the pipeline of Black mental health professionals into the hospital and reimagining ways to serve patients in clinical settings. As chief of the Psychology Department, Sparks piloted and championed a clinical internship program that brought in experts from across the state of Maryland. The program was so successful that interns began serving patients beyond Crownsville's walls, and the application pool included graduate students at prominent Black colleges and universities, including Howard, Morgan State, and Fisk, as well as research institutions such as New York University and Temple University. To this day, the outgrowth of that internship program remains fully accredited, serving patients and providing valuable training for mental health professionals. Dr. Jim Ballard, Vernon Sparks's good friend, has technically retired, but he continues to do talk therapy for forty patients in the Annapolis area. He uses many of the practices he learned from Vernon Sparks.

In memory of and in gratitude to the Holocaust survivors who worked in ways big and small to make Crownsville better:

Ludwig Benedict

Stephen Klinger

Gustav Meinhardt

Hans Meyer

Gisela Morgenstern

Jacob Morgenstern

Hildegard Reissman

Joseph Rosenblatt

Earnestine Sokal

CHAPTER 9

A Bus Ride to Rosewood

IN DECEMBER 1954, FIFTEEN BLACK CHILDREN, TWO TO SIX YEARS old, rode a bus from Crownsville Hospital thirty-five miles north toward Baltimore. As they stared out the window, the trees would have been bare and the many farms that separated their home in Anne Arundel from Owings Mills, Maryland, would have blended together into a sea of brown grass. Turning toward their destination, they would have seen a set of cream-and-gray classical buildings in a U-shaped formation. The little ones didn't know it at the time, but when they stepped off that bus and approached the school's front door, their arrival was the culmination of years of political infighting and administrative feuds. Hundreds of people—742 of them to be exact—had delivered letters to the governor to oppose them. Rosewood's own leadership was shocked to see them standing there. But those fifteen children would walk inside and change their state for good.

Six years earlier, in 1948, a joint House and Senate committee in Maryland made a recommendation: Crownsville should transfer Black "feebleminded" children from its adolescent program to Rosewood, a school that specialized in the care and education of children with a range of diagnoses. Like Crownsville, the school was home to kids with learning disabilities, mental health challenges, or, in some cases, simply nowhere to live. Both had been the subject of shameful investigations.

Though Crownsville was frequently held up as the worst of the worst, one exposé found that Rosewood's administrators had been censoring their patients' mail and trying to keep their students from telling family members what it was really like inside. In the 1940s, a sociologist and conscientious objector named Gordon Zahn alleged that young female patients of Rosewood were permanently placed into the homes of the wealthy and well-connected Marylanders to serve as unpaid domestics.

Rosewood had many failures, but they were consistently regarded to have more space, money, and staff than Crownsville, where children were still often sleeping two to a bed and receiving no formal education. Rosewood was considered to be much more in accordance with medical standards, administrative operations, and educational requirements. Of all institutions in Maryland, Rosewood was the only one fit to take care of children and the only one close enough to reasonably solve Crownsville's chronic overcrowding and staffing problems. Combining their programs would save the state money and help children in crisis. The only issue: Rosewood had always been all white.

Initially, the plan was to transfer about 280 of Crownsville's kids to Rosewood on December 8, 1952. But that date came and went. And Dr. Clifton T. Perkins, the commissioner of mental hygiene who succeeded George Preston, met with his team to let them in on what was going on. The situation was "far hotter" than most of the staff had assumed. In the months leading up to the transfer date, Dr. Perkins had received only one community complaint, and it had come from a landowner near Rosewood who said that he was objecting "because the visiting of colored people to the patients at Rosewood would devaluate the property." But on December 7, the day before the transfer was to begin, he suddenly received a flood of new notices. Parents and unnamed elected officials urged him to pump the brakes. At first, Dr. Perkins pushed the date back by only a few weeks.

What he didn't realize at the time was that white residents—both directly and indirectly connected to Rosewood—had been preparing for war. They hired an attorney. Clifton Perkins was from the far more liberal state of Massachusetts, where he had served as the head of their world-renowned mental health systems. He underestimated Maryland parents—but they knew Yankees well. It didn't take long for them to strategize a new approach, realizing that overt racism might not win a man like Dr. Perkins over.

One hundred and fifty of them formed a new group: the Rosewood Parents Association. The association was similar in structure to some of the "concerned parent" organizations that had historically formed in the United States to push back against integration of public schools or the implementation of a diverse curriculum. They argued that their protest actually wasn't about race—it was about a crisis of resources. They were worried about the well-being of their children at Rosewood, about how additional patients could lead to overcrowding. They gathered one night in January 1953 to formally reject the proposal to move Crownsville patients to Rosewood.

Reporters from the *Washington Star* and the *Washington Post* got access to the parents' meeting. And although most of the parents there that night insisted to reporters that race had nothing to do with it, and that they were worried about space, leaky pipes, and cleanliness, the issue of color appeared to be the elephant in the room. One father, Herbert A. Schiebel, was less shy about his position:

"Dr. Perkins came here roughly three years ago from Massachusetts," he began. "His views as regards race are, I believe, entirely different from those held by the citizens of Maryland. I believe he's a strong believer in civil rights and I believe he's leaning over backward in this thing. We have laws in this state, laws of segregation. This move on the part of Dr. Perkins is only a beginning, an entering wedge. After this the same thing will happen in all state institutions."

That same parent told reporters at the *Star*, "The transfer would not only complicate Rosewood's existing problems, but the admission of colored patients knocks down the racial bars Baltimore has used for generations and would outrage Baltimoreans."

Schiebel accused the commissioner of being too sympathetic to Black patients. His fear wasn't only for the children and families of Rosewood, but for what this might do to the entire balance and culture in Maryland.

More than a year before the Supreme Court would declare racial segregation unconstitutional, Schiebel said aloud what many others in the
room—in the country—were thinking and hoping to hold on to. For
years, white residents had been the first to criticize Crownsville as a failure and a local threat. But when time came to take action on those failures and to find these children a safe, better-funded alternative, these
same communities wanted those patients to believe things weren't bad
enough to warrant help.

The fight only escalated. Two Rosewood parents filed a lawsuit in
Baltimore County on behalf of the parents association, and a judge
moved to block the transfer. One plaintiff argued his child would suffer
through the transfer because it would further degrade Rosewood's facilities. The other said that he had a child on a list waiting to enter Rosewood. If there was a long waiting list for acceptance to Rosewood, why
should patients from Crownsville get to skip the line? Local reporters
kept digging and found that Rosewood actually had 450 vacant beds
and that the wait list had, for the most part, been inactive for years.

Letters from parents kept piling up on the desks of the governor and
Dr. Perkins. Lawmakers chose sides. The Senate sided with Rosewood's
parents seeking to block the transfer, and passed a resolution formally
asking Governor Theodore McKeldin and Dr. Perkins to stop.

Lawmakers in the House, however, took sides with Crownsville's children and blocked the passage of the Senate's resolution. One lawmaker
and Baltimore native Jerome Robinson slammed his colleagues and the
parents association. He called their protests "unreasonable, hysterical,
atrocious, and unsound." Not long after, the Ways and Means Committee issued a report finding what lawmakers had known back in 1948:
children with developmental differences didn't belong in asylums with
adults, Crownsville's facilities were not equal to those at Rosewood, and
the state couldn't afford the millions that it would cost to construct and
hire staff for a separate but equal equivalent on Crownsville's grounds.

Dr. Perkins was struggling to articulate a strategy. But privately, he was
exactly who many of the Rosewood parents suspected he was. He was sympathetic to the children at Crownsville and convinced that the drive behind

the opposition was primarily racism. He believed, according to copies of his correspondence from 1953, that "for the first several days following the original postponement of the transfer (in early December 1952) all objections stated were purely on racial grounds. It was after that period of time that the objectors organized themselves better and tried to shift the stated basis of their objections onto different grounds. They first tried to grasp at the questions of food and clothing and physical care, then they grasped onto the questions of capacity, personnel, and waiting lists. But threaded through all objections which have been advanced against the transfer there still exists the basic filament of discrimination, despite protesting verbalizations to the contrary." Still, for two more years, Dr. Perkins did nothing, unsure of how to move forward against fierce opposition from parents and state senators.

One letter delivered to the governor and his assistant simply stated: "I am writing this letter in protest to sending the colored children from Crownsville Hospital to Rosewood to be mixed with the white children there. Hoping you use your influence in opposing same."

The governor's assistant did not typically respond, but chose to write back to this constituent. "The question is under study by experts. I do not know what their final conclusion will be. I do know it is a question that cannot be decided on the basis of prejudice."

By the end of 1954, the administration at Crownsville had reached the end of their rope. Dr. Morgenstern grew tired of the politics and chose to step down in 1953. The former clinical director of Spring Grove State Hospital, Dr. Arnold H. Eichert, took Morgenstern's place. The staff liked Dr. Eichert, but he didn't have the same patience and talent for coalition building as his predecessor. For years, the lives of his hospital's most vulnerable had been debated in the press and dragged through legislative debates. Even Governor McKeldin and his attorney general were starting to hint to the newspapers that the transfer could restart soon. The Rosewood Parents Association filed new motions in court that December, demanding the state answer more than thirty questions before taking further action. But Dr. Eichert was not interested in waiting.

On December 16, 1954, Dr. Eichert wrote a letter to a probation director in Baltimore, followed by similar notices to the parents of children at Crownsville. "As you have probably read in the newspapers, it has been decided again to proceed with the transfer of the feebleminded children from Crownsville to Rosewood," he told them. "If nothing interferes we expect to move the children from December 27–31." He even sent his letter to Commissioner Perkins for review.

Two days after Christmas, without the knowledge of state leaders or his counterparts at Rosewood, Superintendent Eichert entered the Winterode Building of Crownsville and gathered fifteen Black children. He asked his staff to organize them based on their diagnoses and to choose children who had the best chance of receiving help at Rosewood. They were shepherded onto hospital vehicles by a nurse and a group of attendants.

Eichert had decided that he would rather ask for forgiveness than permission.

The kids climbed into vehicles together. When they finally arrived unannounced on Rosewood's campus, doctors at Rosewood panicked, shocked to see fifteen Black children standing around outside. They knew how it would look to send the children back. They called state officials and colleagues at Crownsville to ask what to do. They realized, according to hospital memos, that once at Rosewood, "the only humane thing to do was to receive those children." They isolated them to test for possible communicable diseases and found rooms to absorb them into the school. Eichert's point was made.

The next day, the *Baltimore Sun* ran a story that read, "The tradition of segregating races in State mental institutions was broken yesterday when 15 Negro children were moved from Crownsville State Hospital to Rosewood Training School."

Dr. Perkins rushed into damage control. He wrote to the secretary of state, insisting he knew nothing of Dr. Eichert's plans. "Neither the Rosewood officials nor I knew of this move until the children were already on their way to Rosewood. I will not burden you with detail, other than to say that a transfer at that time was completely unauthorized," he explained. He warned that it was an unfortunate move that would likely have effects far beyond the hospital system. "I feel that Dr. Eichert erred seriously in this move at that time. I have been led to believe, however, that his error was not malicious—perhaps, careless, at the most... I intend only to reprimand Dr. Eichert for the casual way in which he handled this matter... I might further relieve him of any responsibilities in connection with any further transfers."

Less than a year later, Dr. Eichert quit. He told reporters he was leaving before he even delivered his letter of resignation to Dr. Perkins. Another full year would go by before any additional children from Crownsville were transferred into the superior conditions and school at Rosewood.

It wasn't until November 1962 that the State Board of Health and Mental Hygiene ordered the desegregation of all mental hospitals in Maryland. But with every passing week, more Black men and women took the bus from Annapolis and walked down to Crownsville's campus, where they'd tell the women working in administration how they would love a chance to work with kids or help the elderly. Many of them were determined to be the first in their families to work "professional" jobs—and they succeeded. Desegregation was not the cure to the hospital's problems but rather its new and messy rebirth. As Black staff took on new responsibilities and grew close to their patients, they found themselves bound by the same indifferent, violent, and bureaucratic forces that Eichert had no patience for. The difference, though, was that they couldn't simply walk away.

PART THREE

The Promise of Integration

1945–1970

1945: **1,580 Patients**
1955: **2,719 Patients**
1970: **1,620 Patients**

CHAPTER 10

Love and Broken Promises

O N September 5, 1947, my sixteen-year-old grandmother left Cuba for the first time. Estela Lucrecia Marquetti y Mendieta landed on a Pan American flight carrying with her only one small bag of school clothes and a sum of English words you could count on one hand. She landed in the southern part of the United States with three strikes against her: Black, female, foreign. She made her way to Baltimore and enrolled as a student at Saint Frances Academy, which was at the time an all-girls and all-Black Catholic boarding school.

Those early years in Baltimore were profoundly lonely, yet miraculous. As a teen she had no experiences of best friends, first dates, or school dances, she'd tell me. Her adolescence was spent living in a convent. My grandmother moved in with the Oblate Sisters of Providence that year and stayed with them for free until she finished college. She struggled to make and communicate with friends at school. She spent her time studying, praying, playing card games, and practicing her English with Black women from the oldest order of nuns of African descent in the world. They became her surrogate family, her many mothers in a home far away from her own.

The founder of the order, Mother Mary Lange, had come to Baltimore in the early 1800s from Cuba. What were the odds? A woman who looked like Estela, a descendant of enslaved people from the same narrow island, founding her own order and educational practice during slavery? Here, she was surrounded by women in her image, even if of a different nationality. It was a community and campus full of Black women who had come from all over the country and all over this earth, united in the radical and optimistic belief that little Black girls could be anything and everything. My grandmother was to be no exception. She credited the Sisters' love and protection as the guiding force that helped her heal an aching loneliness, insulate from Baltimore's racism and segregation, and move through the grief of coming of age in heartbreaking circumstances.

Estela was born on the floor of an apartment in Cayo Hueso, which remains a popular Afro-Cuban artist district in central Havana. Her ancestors had been enslaved on sugar plantations in the island's Matanzas province. To this day, my cousins describe themselves as Lucumí—descendants of the Yoruba people. Through a rich oral tradition, generations have been initiated as santeros and santeras into the practice of Santería, blending bits of Roman Catholicism with traditional Yoruban faith.

Americans often think of a whitewashed, uniform Cuban identity, of a nation of people that has somehow skated past the battles over race and justice that we have faced here. That's not the case. My grandmother's mother, Luz Maria, cleaned the homes of wealthy white Cubans while her father, Nicolas, would disappear for weeks at a time. Luz Maria and Nicolas would sometimes go out at night and find they were barred from many white-only spaces. Nicolas would gamble and get wrapped up in petty crime and often fail to bring whatever money he made back home. My grandmother once told me that she had grown accustomed to "weeks with and weeks without." Sometimes she came home to a nuclear family, other weeks Nicolas was off somewhere and there wasn't much to eat.

This was pre-revolution Cuba, and as a select few made money through sugar and corrupt hotels and casinos, many Cubans—especially Black or rural Cubans—were suffering with a lack of public services and a glaring, growing wealth divide. Of course, the United States and other foreign entities owned immense amounts of Cuban land and had their hands in almost everything valuable to the island. To help the family, some of

Estela's siblings started to drop out of school, but Luz Maria and Nicolas made the choice to try and invest in Estela. Nobody knows why they chose her. Estela was simply the child they saved money for, whose suitcase was packed with dreams beyond Havana, and whose feet reached American soil first.

During school breaks, my grandmother would fly from Baltimore back to Havana and find that she had to confront the dysfunction of both her family and her patria—her homeland. When she left home, the last democratically elected president, Ramón Grau, was in power. In 1952, she returned to the start of a coup: U.S.-backed dictator, military sergeant, and former president Fulgencio Batista refused to lose an election and installed himself as the nation's leader once again. This time, he came back ruthless. He crushed, tortured, and jailed his enemies, censored the schools and the press, and allowed for rampant privatization and de facto segregation to disenfranchise Afro-Cubans en masse. In the background of the death and the violence, Havana was becoming a playground for the corrupt, as Batista made the city a safe haven for the American mob in exchange for a cut of their profits. It was "Latin Las Vegas." My grandmother might have felt like she was between two worlds, traveling back and forth from the U.S., but America was also coming to Cuba. Her two worlds were intertwined.

At home, things were crumbling, too. And soon it became clear that my grandmother's beloved older sister, Idalia, was unraveling.

Two months after giving birth to her second child, Idalia began disassociating and hearing voices. The family matriarch, Luz Maria, took on the responsibility and cost of raising Idalia's newborn, and a total of ten people—including siblings, cousins, aunts, and uncles—began coexisting together in a small two-bedroom house in the Lawton neighborhood of Havana. Idalia went in and out of psychosis, experiencing moments of abstraction that made it hard for her to communicate with the outside world. When she came out of crisis, she returned to being the sister and mom she was before, with a warmth and famously big smile restored. She loved and cared for her children as far as her illness allowed. Still, some parts of the family outright rejected Idalia, alarmed and unable to tolerate the instability. Idalia would wander through Havana, go down by the water, and waltz home wired, claiming she had divined a personal message from Fidel Castro. The rebel, the man whose name they heard on the radio and saw in the paper, leading a movement on the other side of the island. He was sending her signs. "He's hiding in the mountains, but he wants me to know he's coming to see me here in Havana soon," she'd say.

It's impossible for me to separate Idalia's delusions from the reality around her. Afro-Cubans in neighboring areas were joining el Movimiento in large numbers, and they were eager for Castro to "see" them, to remake this nation and share it with them. Where there is violence, where there is resistance, there is paranoia. The police, at Batista's orders, were cracking down and killing young militiamen. It's estimated that twenty thousand people on the small island were murdered by the Batista regime, many in horrific and very public executions. And Idalia was right: Batista fled and Fidel did march into Havana in January 1959, marking victory for his revolution and the beginning of the Cuba we know now. But my grandmother's sister Idalia wouldn't get the chance to celebrate or see the man she believed she had spoken to so many times. She was in an asylum.

Apart from her family, Baltimore and the Oblate Sisters of Providence became the center of my grandmother's world. Maryland and the United States were a symbol of calm and possibility for her. Havana came to represent heartbreak, illness, and tumult. Her parents, Luz Maria and Nicolas, suffered harder under the weight of grief. They had lost my grandmother's sister to an illness of the mind, but her brother, Orestes, had also been gravely ill with a strange stomach and bowel disease, and Luz Maria scrambled to get a diagnosis and to afford any medical care. There was no cure. Orestes would lie in bed all day and isolate himself from the rest of the family, growing bitter that he never got a shot at a normal life. No girlfriends, no career, no children of his own. He would die from a disease that was never diagnosed.

Family members had left and joined the revolution. They were focused on building a new Cuba, absorbed by promises of free education, public health, and the eradication of racism. Estela flew back to Baltimore, singularly focused on earning a college degree in chemistry. The Sisters' love and belief in her endured. She became one of the few Black women working in labs at prestigious Johns Hopkins University in the 1950s. As it turned out, order and stability in Baltimore were yet another illusion.

There were parallels between Estela and her sister Idalia. Both women were physically isolated as the rest of the family moved forward together under a single roof. Idalia was coping by constructing a new story of Cuba, one in which she was the close confidant of her nation's new leader. A story in which she was important and wanted. Estela coped by telling herself a story about America that was not true, either. She liked to tell herself that this country was better and more peaceful than being in Cuba because that simplified version of the story soothed her. It eased heartache. It made it easier to leave her hurting family and country behind. But the people who knew her saw the moments when her story would crack, and Estela would become irritable and lash out. She was lonely. I learned so much about storytelling from my grandmother—about how people engage in mythmaking to survive.

The moment Estela fell in love with my grandfather was the moment the bubble she found in Baltimore burst. She met my white Australian grandfather, Edward O'Brien, at a church near Johns Hopkins in 1958. Every Sunday after Mass, Edward would ask Estela if she would like to talk or grab a meal. She always gave a pious "no" and marched home. One day they stepped out of a Mass into the pouring rain. According to Grandpa, Estela turned to Edward and sheepishly asked if she could catch a ride. On paper, the two had very little in common. Edward was born into comfort in rural Toowoomba, the youngest boy from a family with a successful flour company. He was completing his PhD in mechanical engineering. He'd attended private schools his entire life and been a sharpshooter in the Australian military—though he never saw any real action. But she hopped in his car that morning and that was it. Somehow, they built an unbreakable bond.

Maryland was one of the twenty-nine U.S. states that banned interracial marriage and cohabitation. As their relationship progressed, the obstacles piled up. There were countless restaurants where they couldn't eat together, theaters where they couldn't sit together, shops they couldn't safely enter. They were harassed, yelled at, and spit on when they linked arms or held hands together in Baltimore. It was humiliating and scary but Estela was too grown up to retreat behind the walls of a convent. The city she had loved, where she had found a chosen family and constructed a sense of self and safety, proved to be something different. Maryland had rules and racial covenants, and she was breaking them. Some of the dysfunction she so desperately wanted to distance herself from in Cuba had been lurking here all along, too. So the day after Christmas in 1959, Estela and Edward drove to Washington, D.C., to marry and drove right back to Baltimore that night. Their first child—my mother—was born in Baltimore in September 1960. A nurse wrote on my mother's birth certificate that her father—a man completely incapable of getting a tan—was a "negro." Nobody in the family ever asked the hospital why. My mom assumes she did it for Estela's own good. It was another myth that kept my grandmother safe in Baltimore.

According to my grandparents, lawyers with the American Civil Liberties Union reached out to ask if the two of them would be willing to test Maryland's ban on interracial marriage. This was seven years before the Supreme Court struck down state bans on interracial marriage in the groundbreaking *Loving v. Virginia* case. Edward declined to become a test case. He was busy working on his PhD, and worried that if he did take on the case, the toll it would take would destroy their chance to start the big family of their dreams.

In 1961, Edward, Estela, and my mother moved to Long Island. In the summer of 1967, the U.S. Supreme Court ruled that laws banning interracial marriage violated the Equal Protection and Due Process Clauses of the Fourteenth Amendment to the U.S. Constitution. That same year my grandmother gave birth to another child, this time a son whom she named Orestes after her late brother.

Estela never found work as a Black female chemist again. Instead, she became a Spanish teacher. My grandmother poured most of her life into her six children as a strict, rigid, but always wildly passionate mom. She wanted to see each and every child of hers not just succeed, but finish what she had started. She wanted them to shatter the same obstacles she had struggled to sunder. I like to think that they did.

My grandmother's identity straddled different worlds—metaphorically and literally alienating her. She was too hard on herself to ever admit it, but she transcended many of the cultural and social limitations imposed on her. Estela passed away in her bed in New York City in March 2019, forty days after the death of my grandpa. I went to see her days before she passed, and she told me she was on her way out, unable to see the point of living without her best friend. She died surrounded by lots of family. I was there, clutching her right hand. Her nurse, Tracy, told me that when a person dies, the last thing to go is their hearing. She might not have been able to feel me squeeze her hand or kiss her cheek. So I just sat there whispering in her ear, thanking her for every sacrifice she made, every hope and story she held on to for us.

CHAPTER 11

Out of Sight, Out of Mind

A FTER THE END OF THE SECOND WORLD WAR THERE WAS A GROW-ing awareness across the country that mental illness was a burgeoning public health crisis. Americans—like people around the globe—had been living with both real and imagined threats of warfare. Veterans returned home to their families showing signs that they had been physically and mentally disabled by war. Terrifying images of concentration camps and gas chambers had circled the globe.

A new era had begun when American atomic bombs dropped out of the sky on the Japanese cities of Hiroshima and Nagasaki. Now the United States was in the early years of a Cold War and escalating tension with the Soviet Union. Children were practicing how to duck and cover in their classrooms, and people of all ages waited for the signal to find the nearest fallout shelter. Americans were rightly nervous about nuclear weapons, spies, and increased surveillance. International and local news alike offered anxious glimpses into postwar life. A degree of paranoia was baked into the strained social fabric.

At the same time, a rumor spread rapidly across Anne Arundel County: there was a government-funded gas chamber installed on the grounds of Crownsville Hospital, and in the event of an atomic bomb, the state would exterminate its patients to make room for surviving victims. As frightening and unbelievable as those claims sounded, they were bought and spread far enough that the *Washington Post* got hold of them.

In a story published on May 20, 1951, a reporter found the likely source of the rumor: a Crownsville nurse and first aid instructor named Charles F. Nash. Nash had allegedly been telling students in his class at a church hall in Gambrills, Maryland, that Crownsville patients were going to be "disposed of" and that the gas chamber had been built with funds from Congress. He shocked and horrified his students, one of whom wrote a letter to a local commissioner asking, "Is it true these chambers are for inmates who would be considered undesirable in case of an atomic war? Is it true these chambers hold a thousand persons?"

Mrs. James Stewart Martin, a local freelance writer, refused to rest until she got answers. Over the course of weeks, she collected testimony and went to Crownsville superintendent Jacob Morgenstern. She asked him to confirm or deny the speculation.

Morgenstern, a Holocaust survivor, called the claims "fantastic," "silly," and "out of this world." He explained that public tours of the Crownsville campus were underway and had been widely publicized in local papers. One of the four hundred visitors who had attended a recent open house would have surely seen the gas chamber if it existed.

Not to mention, employees at Crownsville knew that the institution had to fight and scrap for enough funding to maintain its core operations—in what world could they afford to construct a gas chamber?

The behavior of Charles Nash, Mrs. Martin, and others involved in the rumor seemed to reflect the Cold War paranoia then sweeping the nation, and the ways in which the horrors of the world were bearing down on everyday people. It was a rumor, a lie with no basis in fact, allegedly perpetrated not by a patient but by a nurse. The lines between reality and imagination, and who was sane and who was insane, were thin. As silly as they seem, those rumors had the potential to cause real harm and to distract from the very real crises that patients at Crownsville had been rioting and crying out for people to listen to.

Rumors notwithstanding, Black people across Maryland were facing systematic violence. People were still sent to Crownsville for the slightest indication of ill health and nonconformity. And after arriving at Crownsville, patients were still crammed into small, overcrowded rooms and given often indifferent treatment.

In the 1950s, there were plenty of authentic horrors at Crownsville and elsewhere.

I'll Be Goddamned, There's the Sky

By the 1950s, psychiatrists and hospital administrators nationwide had been the subject of numerous investigations and scandals. There was growing support for patients and a skepticism about the practice of locking them away in mammoth institutions. At the same time, new medications that could treat psychosis and anxiety were arriving from Europe and inspiring new hope in early trials.

So in 1953, when the National Mental Health Association asked asylums around the country to mail in any shackles or chains they'd previously used, Maryland leaders were eager to take part. It was a public declaration that restraint, fear, and incarceration would have no place in mental hospitals. On April 13 of that year, socialites and politicians, including Governor Theodore McKeldin of Maryland, convened at the McShane Bell Foundry in Baltimore. Together they melted down all of the chains and restraints received during the campaign and turned them into a 300-pound Mental Health Bell. It was a symbol or an aspiration, more than anything, that our society had progressed past a period of coercion and repression.

The excitement may have been premature. Newly hired Black employees at Crownsville were not so hopeful about the latest approaches to treatment.

In 1955, Marie Gough got a job as a patient aide at Crownsville. Marie was a gentle and soft-spoken woman who weighed barely a hundred pounds. On her first day, she was told to report to the A Building at the heart of Crownsville's campus. A Building had been home to more than 1,300 patients, men's and women's wards, an infirmary, staff offices, a

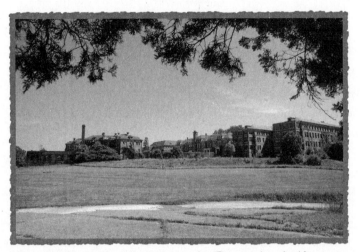

Crownsville Hospital's original campus. At one time, these buildings were
home to thousands of patients. Photo by Cassandra Giraldo.

pharmacy, a clinical laboratory, hydrotherapy wards, and a boiler room.
Marie's first assignment was the men's ward.

Marie didn't know that the A Building was the most notorious on
Crownsville's sprawling campus. There was constant overcrowding, often
no running water, and a stench so strong it would cling to staff's clothing
and hair and never leave no matter how vigorously they tried to wash it off.

As Marie entered the A Building for the first time, she took in the
Georgian pillars and cement steps that marked the entrance. She stepped
through the double doors, and her nerves and excitement gave way to
repulsion. Several patients were slumped over and sprawled across the
cold cement floors. Men were too dazed to sit upright and clearly lying
in their own filth. Marie had little experience working in medicine or
asylums, and she had been thrust into the most challenging, overcrowded
building of them all. Marie started to question what she'd just signed
up for.

She went to meet with her supervisors, two white men who'd worked
there for years. During orientation, she learned that her male patients
needed to eat lunch and dinner, but the A building had no cafeteria large
enough to accommodate them. Each afternoon and evening, Marie was
expected to corral the men and march them from A Building to the
Hugh Young Building.

Marie would walk the men from A building through underground crossways that connected the patients' living areas to the massive U-shaped structure known as the Hugh Young Building, or "HY" as employees called it. Hugh Young was the son of a Confederate brigadier general and one of the physicians on the Lunacy Commission who had pushed for the creation of a Crownsville to relieve Negro patients from the poorhouses and almshouses across the state.

Most of the time, Marie's patients sat around on wooden benches with nothing to do and nobody professional to talk to. She, and everyone else, was completely outnumbered.

Marie's supervisors explained that they only bathed patients at nighttime on Saturdays. She looked around and noticed that there were only a few working toilets and communal showers, and asked, "How do you do the baths?"

"Well, we mix up a bucket of soapy water," one of the men instructed Marie, "and we put the patient in the shower, and we throw the water in on the patient."

Marie, always patient and polite, stood there quietly for a moment.

"No washcloth?" Marie asked.

"No washcloth," her supervisor confirmed.

As part of the original hospital construction plan, many of A Building's facilities were outdated. Most rooms were dark, and some were even outfitted with bars like jail cells. Marie discovered that her colleagues had allowed patients to walk and sit around in soiled clothing for so long that the floors had become covered in matted feces. None of her coworkers had warned her about the excrement she'd been walking in.

Over time, Marie and her friends developed small ways to show the patients affection and care. Armed with rubber dishwashing gloves, they would climb into Crownsville's crumbling communal showers. Instead of throwing the water on patients, they took soap and washcloths and helped those who couldn't bathe themselves. She would cut shoestrings and straw and bring them to the hospital to offer to patients who had been given hospital clothes that were too baggy.

Many of the changes they implemented cost the hospital little beyond a bit of energy and attention to detail. It seemed to Marie as though white staff didn't care how exposed or humiliated the patients looked and felt.

In 2022 I ate lunch with Marie and her friends, many of whom were in their eighties and nineties, and they laughed at the memory of one of Marie's supervisors, who seemed to be a villain to the Black nursing staff. Marie would ask him day after day for permission to take her patients outside. Not off the grounds, just outside the building. Her patients had been stuck moving from dark room to basement to cafeteria and back, and some of the patients housed in A Building hadn't been outside since they were first admitted. They hadn't breathed fresh air or felt the sun against their skin, unless they had been contracted out for work. Marie asked and her supervisor consistently denied her requests, with little or no explanation except that patients might attempt to escape.

One day, he strolled into work announcing: "Marie, you got your wish. You can take the patients outside." Before he could change his mind, Marie rounded up as many patients as possible. The men walked slowly out into a courtyard enclosed by a chain-link fence. One patient, a man named Mr. Bell, walked through the doorway and into the open space.

Mr. Bell stood still. With Marie at his side, he tilted his head all the way back and looked up in awe. "I'll be goddamned," he whispered, "there's the sky."

Seeing Mr. Bell marvel at the clouds and sky brought Marie to tears. This place had taken so much from him. Something about that day stuck with Marie, and she began digging for more information about his life.

Until then, all Marie knew was that Mr. Bell had a British accent. She asked around the hospital and found out that he had been brought to Crownsville by Marie's white supervisor. The supervisor had seen Bell hanging around looking lost in Baltimore one day. After speaking with him, he thought Bell sounded funny and was convinced he was using a fake accent. He put him in a car and brought him to the hospital. Marie said her supervisor childishly bragged about getting twenty-five dollars in cash for the patient delivery.

Former Crownsville employees and even relatives of local law enforcement officers have repeatedly described how they received money in exchange for bringing people to the hospital. It's part of what fueled the nightmares of Black Annapolitans, who used to worry about "night doctors" roaming the streets to bring someone to Crownsville under the cover of darkness. I have not been able to find any evidence of these transactions. There exist no receipts for payment or records describing a program of cash in exchange for patients. But several generations of employees and families shared these stories with me.

Marie learned that Mr. Bell was not, in fact, faking his accent. He was from London. He told her that before coming to the United States, he had been a jockey and raced horses. Marie never found any information that indicated he had a formal diagnosis or had committed a crime. It sounded to her as though Mr. Bell had loitered around and had been stuck at Crownsville for the crime of being a Black man lost in the city with a foreign accent.

More than sixty years after she helped Mr. Bell see the sky again, Marie, now almost ninety, sat with me dressed in her Sunday best. She could still remember every smell, every feeling of A Building. Discussing Mr. Bell still made her cry and visibly shake.

A few years into Marie Gough's career at Crownsville, Joyce and Errol Phillip became two of the newest additions to the Black employee community at Crownsville. Dr. Errol Phillip immigrated to America from Trinidad and Tobago in 1957. Growing up in the capital city, Port of Spain, the Phillip family moved around a lot. In a full house with not enough attention to go around, Errol had raised himself. Inspired by high school peers, he applied to two universities: one in Canada and one in the United States. After being accepted to both, Errol chose the warmer option and enrolled at Howard University. In Washington, D.C., Errol initially pursued a degree in chemistry at the historically Black college. Upon seeing his peers apply to medical school, Errol felt qualified to do the same.

As Errol was settling into his medical studies, his future wife, Joyce, was nearby pursuing a nursing degree. She was born in Xenia in southwestern Ohio, and while Joyce didn't share Errol's island upbringing, they managed to find things in common. Both were from families of six children who had attended Catholic schools for most of their lives. While

Errol was on his road to becoming a doctor, Joyce was a nursing student fulfilling a psychiatric rotation at St. Elizabeths Hospital.

While working in a family practice residency in Flint, Michigan, Errol began searching for a warmer and more welcoming place for his growing family. Michigan was fine but he was tired of being one of only two Black people on staff. By this time, he and Joyce were married with three young children. It was time to find a community. It was in that search that Errol Phillip learned about Crownsville and another Trinidadian doctor with a similar name: Dr. George McKenzie Phillips.

Dr. Phillips was superintendent at Crownsville, the first Black superintendent in the hospital's history. The two men bonded over their love of Trinidad and Tobago and hit it off quickly.

Joyce and Errol took turns driving their family Ford Country Squire station wagon from Flint, Michigan, nine hours south to Crownsville. On June 28, 1968, they moved their three kids into a two-bedroom apartment in Crownsville's employee housing and got to work.

While Errol finished his residency, Joyce took on the role of manager of Crownsville's Psychiatric Research Unit, working with patient records in the Meyer Building. Joyce wasn't always working directly with patients, but she could see their incoming information. "I remember reading a chart of a woman that had been there for a long, long time," Joyce told me. Before Crownsville, this patient had been living on the Eastern Shore. One afternoon, the woman stepped onto a busy road and startled a horse. The horse reared back and frightened its rider, a local white woman. For the "crime" of frightening a white woman on a road, this woman spent years at Crownsville. That was all Joyce could see in documents about her psychiatric history.

Sifting through patient records, Joyce regularly came across similar strange notes. "You'd read stories like that, that had no reason why they should be in Crownsville," Joyce said to me incredulously. "They came to Crownsville and never got out."

Helplessness could set in quickly. Many patients didn't talk—or had never been asked—about their lives before hospitalization. Month after month and year after year of moving between the same dark and dingy buildings took its toll. Former patients have spoken and written about Crownsville the way formerly incarcerated people do of their time in prison. Their instincts, their ways of thinking, their movements are broken down and readjusted to fit this world with its own rules. As time goes on, it becomes harder and harder to feel like part of the outside world, to know they have a place in it if they ever find their way back.

During the pandemic, I would call and Zoom with Faye Belt, leaning on her sharp memory and her many friends to expand my research beyond the institutional records and early oral histories I'd gathered over the last ten years. Sometimes we hit a wall. Generations of patients and employees have died. Those who are still alive are often very elderly. Some had no working landlines or didn't like to answer phone calls. They were not the easiest group to get to click on a Zoom link. But I didn't stop trying. I was desperate to understand what it was like for Black employees to not just enter, but sometimes move into, a place that had once been so openly hostile to them. I wanted to know more about the moral gray areas, the painful decisions, the bizarre balance of power between white employee, Black employee, and Black patient. Finally, as the pandemic eased, it felt safe to pay Faye and her mom, Gertrude, a visit in person.

When I got into town, Faye insisted on picking me up from the Courtyard by Marriott on Riva Road. She wanted to show me some of her spots in Annapolis and make sure that I had great food. I had seen most of Annapolis before, and I was a bit nervous—I had a lot of work to do and sources to meet with.

I gave in. For three days, I spent almost every waking minute with her. I saw the hospital and the shoreline of the Chesapeake through her. One afternoon, she took me to her mother's home, the house that her dad, Freddy, built, and she opened the door. All Faye told me was that we'd have some lunch and lemonade with a few people she wanted me to meet. She led me through the kitchen to a dining room at the back of the house. There was Joyce Phillip, and a dozen other former Crownsville employees. Many of them I had already tried, and failed, to locate and interview. Now here they were, crowded around a dining room table, telling me to get to it and turn on my recorder.

Two of them—Thelma Lovelace and Dorothea McCullers—brought along their old Crownsville Hospital employee identification badges. Former nursing director Betty Hawkins had an entire packet of patient poems and drawings and photographs for me to copy. Some of them had jotted down their memories or their former colleagues' names on notepads. I realized that Faye had made calls on my behalf and had even made in-person visits to urge some people to make time for me. She had gone out of her way to bring generations of Crownsville together for me and this book.

From there, the memories started flowing. Donald Williams, a licensed practical nurse who worked in the Hugh Young Building, wanted me to understand that there was a Crownsville before Black staff and a Crownsville after. When he first started, he was disturbed by how filthy Crownsville was. Most of the white staff he worked with hailed from Virginia and other states farther south, and they refused to do any housekeeping or laundry for their Black patients. New Black hires had to clean the buildings.

Their arrival changed the atmosphere, Donald said. He noticed that the patients started to have more trust and comfort with staff. Donald began attending subsidized hospital courses where he learned to deliver medication to patients under supervision. Once he received the necessary certifications, Donald was able to transfer to the Meyer Building, excited by the constant opportunities to improve and work with different patient populations. Crownsville gave his family stability and opportunity, just as it had for the Belt family. But the more he knew, the more concerned him about Crownsville.

First, there were the abysmal records. On the forensic unit working with court-committed patients, Donald said he often received charts for patients with little or no information on them. There was nothing to guide nurses and other medical staff in their care. Donald's comments reminded me of a previous visit to Annapolis in 2014, when I received permission to access records at Maryland State Archives that included the Patient Master Index, a recordkeeping system of detailed two-sided cards, each representing a different patient's medical history at the asylum. These cards were intended to keep information about the patient: place of birth, home address, age, close contacts, diagnoses over time, date of discharge or death, cause of death, burial place, and more. But more often than not, the surviving patient cards I saw were incomplete. There was another category of records called the "Death and Discharge Summary" that I was not allowed to see, and which I have been told contains more information.

Clinical notes often privilege the provider's point of view and enforce hierarchies and power. Doctors and nurses were the ones who decided what was valuable information and what would constitute the story of patients' lives behind Crownsville's walls. And of course, to make matters more fraught, most of the clinical-level staff were white people writing about Black patients in this period. Patient records and monthly hospital reports from the 1950s and early '60s, at least those found or made available to me and other researchers, suggest that Crownsville was better equipped for production and industrial maintenance than it was outfitted for therapy and treatment. By neglecting almost all personal and contextual information about their patients and doing little to preserve even a doctor's account of clinical encounters, the hospital erased the patients' humanity.

Then, Donald realized that a lot of the patients he met were admitted only because county jails were too full. Even when Donald didn't know a patient's complete backstory, he was often baffled by how healthy and "normal" they were. "They could talk as well as I could," he said. "They knew about history. They knew about what's going on in the world." He'd ask himself, "Why the hell are they here?"

As Donald spoke, another LPN, Barbara Shank, hummed in agreement. In her work, she saw many patients picked up and brought to Crownsville under the guise of anti-vagrancy laws. Patients had gotten drunk in public or had slept on the street, and woke up at Crownsville.

Betty Hawkins recalled going through patient files one day and reading about someone who was admitted after stealing a small soda. She did what she could to get patients like that released. One afternoon, a patient in the HY Building approached one of her student interns in desperation. For some time, this patient had been begging for any and everyone to listen. He said he didn't belong in an asylum, and he had told this to Crownsville staff and even affiliate nurses who traveled in from nearby cities, but no one had taken him seriously. The patient gave this student a phone number and the address of his brother, who he said lived in Washington, D.C. "Please, give them a call," he begged.

The student went to Betty Hawkins. "Let's call him right now," Betty said. Everything the patient said was true. His brother had been looking for him for years and had no idea where he was. He thought his brother had been kidnapped or killed, but he was just waiting around at Crownsville the entire time. Betty notified the necessary administrators of the "mix-up" and got him out. That patient wasn't the only one. Another patient Betty worked with had been at the hospital for twenty-seven years. Betty, worried about how isolated this patient had become, contacted their relatives in Baltimore. The family was in shock. They, too, had no idea their loved one was there. They immediately drove over to the hospital to bring him home. For twenty-seven years, a Baltimore family had assumed the worst.

The historical record confirms much of what the employees described. In a 1953 article, "Crowding of Youths at Crownsville Told," the chief supervisor of social work at Crownsville, Gwendolyn Lee, noted that some of the overflowing patient population was not arriving of its own will. The hospital received "too many teenagers with no hope," she said, and many of them arrived by force. Lee argued that there was "too large a percentage of cases where people are picked up off the street and taken to Crownsville without the knowledge of relatives... Less than 2% of the mentally ill are brought by relatives."

Lying just off the hospital grounds, Gertrude Belt's home had become a haven and escape for Black staff and patients. In this same living room where I now sat, patients had come over for playdates when Faye was little. They sang gospel music with her siblings and played with toys. Faye didn't realize it at the time, but her mom was trying to give young female patients somewhere to go and a family to connect with. Sometimes she offered them a home-cooked meal, and other times Gertrude allowed them to sleep over or asked the older adolescent girls to babysit Faye.

Over the years, Crownsville had developed into a dumping ground—a place that seemed to swallow the undesired, poor, and nonconforming Black residents of Maryland and, at times, deny them fundamental human rights. Black employees, many of whom came from the same neighborhoods and conditions as their patients, found themselves working under impossible and ethically compromising conditions. They were not always confident that their work was enough to outweigh the harm, but the alternative—a return to the days of a white-only professional staff—seemed far worse.

Lost to the Hospital

Summers in Annapolis are notoriously muggy. The sun and mosquitoes take turns clinging to your skin. Breezes drifting inland from the bay are welcome to anyone not already cooling off in the water. Some families laze on the beach or on boats in the bay, while others spend the afternoons looking for the best Maryland blue crabs swimming in the rivers.

All of the beauty of a summer in Maryland belied a painful, precarious truth. Summer fun was segregated. Jewish families were barred from certain beaches and establishments, while Black families had to be especially careful about where they spent their time together. For so many in the fifties and sixties, Carr's Beach, a private beach venue and resort located just south of Annapolis, was the beginning and the end of summer. One of a few where those months were free of racial prejudice. Originally owned by the daughter of a former slave, Elizabeth Carr Smith, the Carr's Beach waterfront restaurants and venues were raucous from day to night. Teenage couples found dark corners, and adults joined in jitterbug dance competitions. Thousands of people would cram into a pavilion where everyone from Billie Holiday to Otis Redding and James Brown graced the summer stage.

It was in this environment—the warmth, the water, the social unrest—that Rodney Barnes was born in Annapolis in the 1970s. His grandmother's small home was in a historic Black neighborhood right on the water. The kind of close-knit community that didn't need an excuse for a picnic, especially in the summertime. Any holiday or clear-skies forecast was a good enough reason to convene in a friend's or family member's backyard.

On one summer afternoon, when Rodney was about seven years old, half the neighborhood gathered for a barbecue. Trays of food covered several tables. Music filled the air, interrupted only by the laughter and loud conversation of some of the adults. Rodney, like all the other cousins and neighbors his age, had been left to his own devices. They crawled under plastic tables and wrestled in the grass.

A loud scream jolted them out of a game of make-believe. Rodney stopped and looked up to see his aunt.

He remembers thinking, *My aunt isn't acting the way grown-ups are supposed to act.* She began sprinting back and forth, shouting at the top of her lungs. Everyone fell quiet, watching her. Rodney doesn't remember what she said or who she was shouting for, but he remembers the way her screams pierced through that summer afternoon.

For much of his little life, Rodney had heard them all use the words. "She's a little *off.*" "She's *crazy.*" Rodney's family didn't talk about grown folks' business or feelings in front of the kids. Children were seen but not often heard from. But for these few moments, a family truth seemed to be right there at the surface, confronting all of them, demanding some kind of response.

Later that afternoon, Rodney overheard an adult say that she was being sent to Crownsville. No one followed up with him or the other cousins to explain what had happened to her. In a matter of minutes on a summer afternoon, Rodney lost his aunt to Crownsville Hospital. Nobody spoke of her, nobody visited her. He never saw her again.

It's impossible to quantify how many Black children lost or lost track of parents, aunts, uncles, and friends to the hospital. In fact, it took decades for Rodney to come to terms with his aunt's story. A lot of silence insulated him from the truth of what happened to her.

For most of his life, mental illness and trauma weren't discussed. Not in the way he is now able to name it. Back then, if someone was depressed, they were told it was a bad mood. To fix the depression, that person only needed to go outside and play or be a man. There was an unsaid expectation for that person to walk it off, as everyone else did with the things that tormented them. People with mental health challenges were people to stay away from or to pity. Rodney didn't feel a lot of empathy for people like his aunt.

While Rodney didn't always have the language to describe what was shifting around him, he was observant. As the son of a schoolteacher, he spent countless hours alone reading the books and the *Ebony* and *Jet* magazines his mother left lying around. Occasionally, he'd walk over to the local theater and watch movies about a world beyond Annapolis.

Rodney was a Black boy coming of age in an America where integration was still a new and fragile thing. Rodney's grandmother worked at the homes of white families as a domestic. Each morning, Rodney attended school with white children, and each afternoon, he joined his grandmother, who was helping to raise him in his father's absence. He'd often make it home first and wait around on his best behavior until his grandmother was relieved of her duties. All of this time alone gave Rodney the chance to think, eavesdrop, and brood. It was in this way that Rodney came to know more about the asylum.

There was the Crownsville that Rodney knew through the Black women in his life. Almost every adult Black woman he knew had worked a stint as a nurse at Crownsville. Then, there was the communal understanding of Crownsville that Rodney gathered through Black Annapolis at large. From an early age, Rodney heard whispers of a boogeyman facility. In these stories, people were scooped up for being in the wrong place at the wrong time. If a fight broke out at Carr's Beach and the jail was too full, you were sent to Crownsville. If you were young and unsupervised late at night, you were taken to Crownsville. He knew about Janice Hayes-Williams's uncle, George Phelps Jr., and how he would threaten "bad kids" with a trip to Crownsville.

In his mind, Crownsville was a place you didn't want to go. A prison for crazy people or a punishment for derelicts. Rodney never really associated the hospital with mental illness or even treatment. So much so that he struggles to call the people sent to Crownsville "patients." Young

Rodney heard stories and rumors, and it all seemed to confirm a larger suspicion he had of his hometown. The deck was stacked against his people.

It has been a long time since Rodney was that little boy at the summer barbecue. Today, Rodney is an entertainment industry veteran and prolific comic book writer. He's the brains and pen behind shows like *The Boondocks*, HBO's *Winning Time*, and classics like *My Wife and Kids* and *Everybody Hates Chris*. Rodney has made a living building new stories and worlds for Black people, and his writing has become a way for him to wrestle with and understand America.

Annapolis and Crownsville reshaped the way Rodney views mental illness, and turned him into someone who likes to talk openly about depression and anxiety. His view is that people are not the problem. Rodney has learned not to judge the way people deal with their emotions. When developing a character or writing a script, Rodney tries to be gentle—even with his antagonists.

Looking inward, he has seen the ways anxiety and depression have shown up in his adult relationships. Adulthood became a mirror for what he experienced and saw go unaddressed as a child. A successful career in Hollywood couldn't save him from his childhood experiences.

Decades after his aunt's disappearance into Crownsville, Rodney paid a visit to the hospital's grounds. He walked around, trying to imagine what his aunt's life might have been like.

Rodney has not made an effort to find out what happened to his aunt or to request her records from the state. When I asked why, he hesitated. "There's so many folks in my family who've gone through so much. It opens the door to so many things. Virtually everyone in my family, to lesser or greater degrees, has had a brush with some type of exploitation, trauma, something from the system that haunted them into their adult lives. Going down that rabbit hole..." His voice lowered. "Maybe at some point I will."

In 1955, the *Baltimore Afro-American* reported that the Eastern Shore State Hospital for the mentally ill had no intention of opening its doors to help Crownsville, even though it had forty vacant beds. Crownsville, at the time, had 2,445 patients crowded into space that could only accommodate 1,500. There were over 600 patients in Crownsville from the Eastern Shore, a peninsula area notorious among Black residents for its cross burnings and for the lynchings of George Armwood and Matthew Williams. Despite having extra space and a geographic advantage, the hospital was unwilling to accommodate Crownsville patients who had been residents and taxpayers in its counties. White Marylanders were not only indifferent to the therapeutic circumstances for Crownsville patients, but preferred that the patients stay as far away as possible in a well-isolated establishment.

These patterns were set long before people like Paul Lurz or Sarah Maddox arrived, but it was agonizing for them to watch the hospital become a facility for people the state had no plan to help and nowhere else to send. Even though they could recognize the greater social and systemic factors at fault, they couldn't help but feel personally responsible.

In December of the following year, Dr. Ralph Meng, Crownsville's superintendent, penned a letter that has been preserved at the Maryland State Archives. He wrote to a Johns Hopkins Hospital social worker, worried about these same patterns. Dr. Meng was concerned that local agencies were not willing to accept their obligation to serve the patients who were ready for discharge back into the community. He estimated "that about 40% of our patients could be handled without hospitalization if anybody made an effort to do so."

Almost half a century into its existence, Crownsville was a place that mixed constant striving and suffering. A May 1957 *Baltimore Afro-American* article reported on the resignation of Superintendent Ralph Meng after just one year in his role as the hospital leader. According to the piece, Meng "deserted in despair." Even with the best of intentions, retaining quality leadership was proving near impossible. Plagued by low funding and negative public perception, the hospital seemed incapable of escaping its legacy of systematic racism. "Segregation was expensive," the article read, "and the people who suffer most when budgets are cut are the patients in the Jim Crow institution."

The Boy from the Old Fourth Ward

Before assuming his role as Crownsville's director of social work, Paul Lurz worked in the adolescent ward. Young, orphaned children often ended up there when social services couldn't—or wouldn't—place them in homes. It should have been the job of county social services departments, but those agencies had backlogs. Patients in the adolescent ward were divided into small groups among staff like Paul. Each child was assigned to a therapist or other medical professional who became responsible for them.

Paul worked with a group of about seven kids. Most of the children attended public school, but their lives outside of the classroom revolved around Crownsville. He saw them each day before class and was there to greet them when they got off the bus and returned to the hospital.

Paul saw firsthand that many of them did not have severe mental illnesses. Some had developmental delays or learning disabilities. Others had depression and were struggling with resentment and anger. But a lot of kids on the adolescent ward simply wanted to be adopted. In Paul's view, an asylum overflowing with adults—some mentally ill, some accused of crimes, many discarded—was no place for a child who was searching for a guardian.

Hospital staff called extended family members and tried to cozy up to agencies to see what they could do. But people simply did not want kids from Crownsville. Paul's close friend and the first Black nurse at the hospital, Sarah Maddox, would joke that he was always begging her to foster one of the children. And she did. Sarah Maddox and her mother fostered adolescents that Paul couldn't place elsewhere. One was a teenage girl who Sarah raised as her own after constant refusals by social service placement agencies. Sarah took in another young man until he was ready to go off to college.

In the mid-1960s, Paul worked closely with two teenage boys in particular: one white and one Black. Around 1963, Crownsville—like all publicly run facilities—became required by law to admit patients of all races, pushing the patient population toward the kind of demographic changes seen among the staff. Between December 1962 and December

1967, Crownsville's patient population went from being entirely nonwhite to approximately 70 percent Black. According to hospital records from 1968, the patient population remained majority Black in large part because twice as many Black people were being admitted to the system as white people. Still, this was supposed to mark a new era in the hospital's reputation and acceptance throughout Maryland.

The two teenage boys were around the same age and had been inseparable friends since they first arrived at Crownsville. They did everything together, and Paul was the closest thing to a guardian these boys had. On school picture day, Paul would pay out of pocket for their school photos. The boys would race back to the hospital at the end of the day, smiling ear to ear. Instead of giving copies out to parents, aunts, uncles, and grandparents, the boys made sure their favorite staff members received their 4 × 6 headshots. Paul got a set, as did Sarah Maddox and a few others.

Paul loved his kids but he also wanted more for them. After being effectively left at Crownsville as vulnerable children, all these two had was each other. Paul wanted to do everything he could to keep them together. State agencies hadn't been able to place them, but perhaps a private organization could.

Paul called up a religious agency in Baltimore to gauge their interest. He spoke with a polite social worker over the phone and gave her some background on the boys, who had always been a delight to have at the hospital. "Of course we'll see them," she told Paul. "Bring them out."

Everyone was thrilled. Staff wanted the boys to put their best foot forward for their interview with the social worker. For days, the boys practiced being as polite as possible to leave a strong first impression. They rehearsed answers to questions they might be asked about their past or education. On the morning of the boys' interview, nurses came to find them. They cleaned the boys up and gave them the best clothing from storage. They made sure everything fit.

When it was time to go, Paul didn't want to risk arriving in one of the banged-up vehicles the hospital set aside for the social workers, so he piled the excited and well-groomed boys into his personal car.

The three made the trek to the agency office and were ushered into a waiting room. Paul was the first to be interviewed, and he instructed the boys to sit quietly while he and the social worker chatted. The social worker seemed just as compassionate as she sounded on the phone, and Paul was feeling hopeful.

But before their conversation had ended, the agency director stormed in. "Why are you here?" he shouted at Paul. Before Paul could explain or tell him about the boys, the director spoke over him. "How could you even think we would take *these* kids?"

Paul was stunned. This man hadn't even laid eyes on them. "It was like I was insane for bringing them here," he recalled. He wracked his brain for some kind of answer or explanation. He assumed it was prejudice. Crownsville had slowly begun integrating its patient population, beginning with the adolescent program, but it was still known as the "Negro" hospital and most of the wards were still entirely Black. The only saving grace, it seemed, was that this man hadn't seen the one white boy. Paul could try again to keep the two best friends together.

The director kicked Paul out of his office. The social worker walked quietly behind Paul and waited until the director was out of earshot. She apologized profusely and told him she was embarrassed by her boss's actions.

Paul told the boys to collect their things and prepare to leave. They kept asking him why their visit had ended so abruptly, why they didn't even get the chance to share any of the answers they had spent days rehearsing. Paul didn't have the strength to tell them the truth.

Thankfully, they hadn't heard the director's words for themselves. Paul mumbled something about how it was not working out and there were actually no spots available.

The two boys were eventually placed in homes, though not together and not with any of their biological families.

Decades after Paul first helped them, many of the former children of Crownsville remembered him and stayed in touch. They wrote to him with updates on their lives, and he'd tell them about his hobbies, too. Paul always thought of himself as progressive and well informed, but he had been shocked by the callousness of the system. It was the small success stories, the moments when he was able to reconnect children with their families or find them good local schools to attend, that reassured Paul of his path.

In 1965, Superintendent George McKenzie Phillips, the first Black man to lead any Maryland hospital, moved onto the Crownsville campus and began to centralize children into one unified ward within the Winterode Building. The "building" was really a collection of structures huddled around one another. Built in 1942, the Winterode complex stood northwest of the central campus buildings and was separated from them by the old morgue and a pump house. The Winterode Building had a dining room with expansive windows looking out at the rest of the grounds. It was beautiful on the outside, where there were covered outdoor walkways that connected every space. Inside was not so nice. It had deteriorated. And there was a large, putrid garbage room that struggled to contain the waste of the three buildings in the complex.

At the time, judges would sometimes send kids who got in trouble to Crownsville as punishment. If the adolescent ward was too full, the kids would end up living out on adult wards. Children and teenagers were often scattered across the hospital, depending on when and why they were admitted. Getting placed into rooms with patients much older and bigger than they were opened some of the kids up to abuse and beatings. Paul and his colleagues would routinely make rounds of the hospital to try and find these children and bring them back to his team in the Winterode Building.

In October 1966, a fifteen-year-old Black boy named John arrived at Crownsville. His family lived down in the Old Fourth Ward in Annapolis, a historic Black neighborhood not far from the water. They brought him to the hospital that fall, after John showed signs of becoming detached and quiet. The hospital admitted John and housed him in an adult ward. Then he met Paul Lurz.

John was kind and easy to like, beloved by staff and patients from the moment he arrived. Paul was accustomed to working with young patients who arrived rightfully suspicious and angry, who would lash out as they struggled to adjust to life in a strange and clinical place. John was not like that. He was calm. But as time went on, he became increasingly withdrawn. He would hardly eat and rarely wanted to leave his bed. To Paul, it appeared John was lost and depressed. John's body was here. He was present and awake. But one by one, the illness was severing his connections to everything that kept him rooted *here*. With each day, more of John—the real John—was slipping away.

Everyone living in the brick row houses on Obery Court in the Old Fourth Ward knew John and his family. His father, John Sr., was a maintenance man for the housing authority, and a talented drummer who led the Annapolis Drum and Bugle Corps. Every family that lived along their street depended on one another. They went to school together, bought food from each other, and worked in the same places. The younger John grew up running around the neighborhood with all the local kids, goofing off near the train tracks that ran right behind their houses, and occasionally getting chastised for covering someone's house with rolls of toilet paper. Mostly, he loved to pick berries and spend his afternoons fishing with friends like Nick Carter. Nick remembers John as someone who was always waiting outside, eager to play games with the other boys. It seemed to Nick, who was about two years older, like John was searching for acceptance and affection he wasn't getting at home.

The neighborhood kids respected John's father. But everyone knew he was hard on his son. Nothing the younger John did seemed to be good enough. John learned how to play the snare drum just like his dad, and he pushed himself at baseball and football. The neighborhood kids all sensed that John Sr. resented him anyway. Both John and his father were only about five feet tall, and Nick remembers how John Sr. would constantly comment on his son's weight and size, like he was repulsed by his own reflection.

In his early teens, John started to get into a little trouble. He'd throw rocks and bricks into neighbors' windows and withdraw from his friends for days at a time. Whenever John lost a football game or made a mistake, Nick would watch as his friend broke down. "He needed to be wanted, you know. And that's hard to take," Nick told me. "He was just erratic…

it was like flashes, he would be himself and then all of a sudden turn into another totally different person."

Nick remembers the last time he saw his friend. Nick and John were standing on the corner of Washington and Clay Street, joking around. John looked and sounded like his old self again. He was playing around, challenging Nick to one last race down the block to prove who was the fastest. Nick was planning to join the Marine Corps soon, and he chuckled, telling John he was getting too old now for their childhood games.

Next thing Nick knew, John had disappeared.

One day when Nick was back home, he walked over to his friend's old house and saw John Sr. outside. "Where's JR?" he asked.

"He gone," John Sr. replied curtly.

That winter at Crownsville, the staff who worked with John were beginning to worry for his survival. Paul and a group of nurses urged the doctors in charge of his care plan to do more. But the psychiatrist assigned to John had another theory. The psychiatrist believed that John's refusal to eat was proof of "attention-seeking behavior." He told the staff they had to ignore John—he believed that the only way his eating would return to normal was if the staff didn't play into his selfish act.

Depression can look like selfishness. And in the 1950s and '60s, we did not know as much about depression as we do now. Depression was thought to be rare; anxiety, stress, and neuroses were the psychiatric profession's focus at the time. Few were interested in depression's manifestations in communities of color. Still, a psychiatrist who worked at Crownsville Hospital would have seen and lived beside thousands of patients. Paul, who is not a doctor, had seen children whose pain had manifested as isolation, irritability, anger, exhaustion, self-hatred. To him, there was no doubt John needed someone to help lift him out of the fog.

The nursing staff ignored the doctor's orders and continued to worry about John. They would come by his bed to check on him frequently and try to get him to finish his food. One nurse would try to sneak John snacks at night.

Days later, the psychiatrist was back, annoyed with his colleagues. As the doctor in charge, he ordered that John be kept in a chair and surrounded by a set of opaque screens. The screens, he argued, would block the nurses' view of John so that they couldn't be moved or taken in by his expressions. Of course, this only isolated him even further. John stopped eating altogether.

After days of this, John was transferred to the Medical Surgical Building, where he died. I obtained a copy of John's death certificate, and it listed his cause of death as "hypostatic pneumonia." This is not the pneumonia many are familiar with; it is a medical term for congestion, fluid, and blood stagnant in the lungs and chest cavity. It typically affects animals or the elderly who have been left lying down so weak they're unable to move or reposition their body. There was no peer review of the psychiatrist's treatment decisions. As far as Paul knows, nobody was punished for what happened to John, although some of the staff stopped speaking with the doctor in charge.

Paul couldn't process the news. John died in February 1967, having stayed at the hospital for only four months. Paul and the nursing staff who had tried so hard to give John comfort were devastated.

John's mother invited them to attend his homegoing at a nearby Black church. Paul remembers the day was gray and cold. What he remembers most are the sounds of John's family crying. The way they mourned with their entire bodies. Toward the end of the service, John's shrunken body lay still in the coffin as the undertaker wheeled him slowly past the family for a final look. A church attendant hurried from one row to another tending to the mourners. Suddenly, John's mother threw herself onto the casket, holding tight to her son's body.

Watching all of this and listening to the sounds of wailing fill the sanctuary, Paul began to tremble. His own emotions overwhelmed him. He thought he might faint.

A woman seated next to him turned to him with a knowing look: "You can't keep so much feeling bottled up." He had been granted permission. Tears streamed down Paul's face as the woman assured him, "It's okay to cry, to shout it out." There in that church, Paul learned what it was to grieve loudly and publicly. What it meant to bear witness to a community's loss and anger.

Back on the Old Fourth Ward, Nick was struggling to get answers from his own community. Again, he tried to ask John Sr. where his friend had gone. Each time, he heard some variation of "He's gone for a while. We expect him back." Nick knew better than to question his elders, but he also sensed someone was keeping the truth from him. John Sr.'s moods seemed even heavier than before, and Nick could see that he had started drinking more openly. Rumors began to circulate that John had been sick, that he had ended up at Crownsville. Nick, who had grown up afraid of the hospital, knew many of the women in the community had started to work there. And yet, none of them would tell him that that was where his friend had gone. Nobody told him when John died, and nobody invited him to the funeral.

It was jarring just how quickly life at Crownsville and on the ward returned to its daily routine with patients, activities, therapy, and laughter in the lunchroom. John's death rendered Paul vulnerable—and for the first time, he started to doubt his life's purpose and the impact he could have. Paul had come to Crownsville to do the right thing for children, to materially improve their lives and relationships. And yet he had been adjacent to the harm done to John. He had been a witness. It was the doctor who had made the decisions and ignored the clear warning signs, but it was Paul and the nurses who were left wracked with guilt. Paul couldn't grasp how a fifteen-year-old could enter Crownsville and be buried a few months later.

John was laid to rest at Brewer Hill, the city's oldest Black, segregated cemetery. To this day, the grass grows wildly high, and the tombstones tilt, where seven thousand people, including former slaves, relatives of Harriet Tubman, a founder of the Alpha Kappa Alpha sorority, and descendants of John Quincy Adams, rest. Black Annapolitans such as historians and lifelong residents Carl Snowden and Janice Hayes-Williams continue to fight for the cemetery's restoration and upkeep.

Records and oral history show that some of the doctors, directors, and staff at Crownsville, and much of the state leadership responsible for the hospital's funding and care, directly and knowingly harmed patients.

They also show that the dysfunction and stigma associated with the hospital made it easier for them to carry out this harm. But this hospital was not a sensational snake pit, full of caricatures instead of people. In my research, I've found that most of the employees—especially the longtime ones—entered Crownsville desperately trying to make it better. They had no illusions about how difficult that would be in a system as large as the one serving the whole state of Maryland. But they loved their patients, and they knew their patients. Many of the Black employees had grown up on the same block or had taken the bus to school with the people who then ended up in their care.

They were human, and the longer they worked there, the more often they found themselves in situations that forced them to ask the same questions over and over again. Is it worth it, doing incremental good in an imperfect system? Can you be a good person and work somewhere where something like this happens?

Paul and many of the employees at Crownsville remind me of a story I grew up hearing from the Caribbean side of my family. One of my aunts in particular loved the Starfish Story. Legend has it that a young Black boy—in Haiti or Cuba or the Dominican Republic, you choose—is walking along a beach that is littered with starfish. Thousands upon thousands of starfish have washed up onto the shore following a terrible storm and they are helpless, dehydrating in the sun. So the little boy begins picking the starfish up one by one and throwing them back into their home in the water. Other people at the beach look at the boy, laugh, and call him naive. One person approaches him and tells him bluntly, "Give up. It makes no difference. You'll never be able to save all of these starfish." The boy pauses for a second.

He looks up, then leans back down to toss another starfish into the sea. "It makes a difference for that one."

Many of the people of Crownsville decided that it was better to throw as many starfish back into the ocean as they could rather than abandon them all on the shore.

CHAPTER 12

Medical and Surgical

A poem by a Crownsville patient who went by the pseudonym Mr. New Unit, written in April 1952:

If you get sick against your will
They will bring you to Crownsville
But if you're a lucky so-and-so
It won't be long before you go

The doctors keep you until—
And there you'll stay in Crownsville
And if they don't make up their mind
You'll stay there for a long, long time

But when it's time for you to go
You and everybody will know
And your mission you'll fulfill
Then you can leave Crownsville

But some day in the sweet by and by
You won't have to stay there
Until you die

Just trust in God and you can depend
He will bring things to an end.

Lucile Elsie Pleasant, known as Elsie Lacks, delivered herself in 1940. Her mother, Henrietta Lacks, went into labor in the former slave home-house where generations of family had been born. As her father, Day, rushed to summon the midwife, Elsie could not wait another second to see the world. As author Rebecca Skloot told it in *The Immortal Life of Henrietta Lacks*, Henrietta's newborn shot out and hit her fragile skull on the floor. Everyone in the family agreed that Elsie was beautiful and looked so much like her mom. But Elsie would always be different—from her family and most people in their community. She didn't speak and couldn't hear. She communicated through murmurs and chirps. When not running through the grass and playing with farm animals, Elsie often sat in silence.

Skloot discovered Elsie's story as she embarked on a decade-long retracing of Henrietta Lacks's life with Deborah, Henrietta's daughter and Elsie's younger sister. Her work uncovered the unbelievable story behind the tissue that doctors at Johns Hopkins extracted from Elsie's mother and used without her consent to develop an immortal, and seemingly invaluable, human cell line, known as HeLa. But as her mother's cells were transformed into billion-dollar drugs and vaccines, Elsie was at Crownsville. The evidence suggests she was used by science, too.

Elsie was diagnosed with cerebral palsy, epilepsy, and "idiocy." As she grew older, she grew more curious and boisterous. According to Skloot, everyone assumed it was her birth that had kept her mind "like an infant's." After a few clumsy accidents that left Elsie's skin bruised and burned, it was clear she needed constant supervision—or healing. Henrietta and Day would drive Elsie to see preachers in tents, and these men would try to perform their miracles. None of them worked.

As Elsie's condition only worsened, Henrietta and Day struggled to manage. Before, Henrietta would soothe her daughter by combing her curls or rocking her. But now, Elsie was having more frequent outbursts. Doctors told Henrietta and Day that sending Elsie away to a hospital was best for everyone.

Crownsville was a long way away for the Lacks family, and the hospital wasn't the easiest to access by public transport. Nevertheless, for the first year or two that Elsie was there, Henrietta visited her every week.

She boarded the train from Baltimore and waited patiently in the hospital's visitation room to see her daughter. When Elsie arrived, she and Henrietta would snuggle. They'd fall into their old routines, combing and playing with one another's hair.

Elsie was ten years old when she arrived at Crownsville. She was only fifteen when she died there alone.

༄

Elsie arrived at Crownsville as a small number of Black aides and nurses were starting to get their feet in the door. In most cases, they had come from families just like Elsie's. They were working to support children and trying to find a way to get along with white colleagues who they knew didn't really want them there. They all wanted something better.

What they likely didn't know at the time was that the field they were entering was trying to rapidly professionalize, even as its leaders and practitioners were scrambling in the dark. Every early development and disease categorization, and every plan for how to treat a child like Elsie, was being touted as a great advancement. In truth, they were treating symptoms, and they knew next to nothing about the origins of mental illness and distress.

That didn't stop the pressure to construct a veneer of competence. Psychiatrists and psychologists across the country started to gather more frequently at conferences and symposiums. Growing numbers opened private practices and started advertising treatments for the anxieties and disturbances affecting the upper classes. Maryland's health officials began performing mandatory inspections of every asylum, and set statewide goals to match the professional recommendations from national organizations like the American Psychiatric Association (APA).

In the midst of this push, in the fall of 1954, the APA notified Superintendent Arnold Eichert that Crownsville failed to meet basic standards and would not be approved for accreditation. The APA echoed what patients and their families had been saying for years: Crownsville was severely overcrowded and understaffed.

The APA made their decision after extensive tours of Crownsville's facilities, interviews with staff, and supervision of their services. Unsurprisingly, inspectors found wards brimming with untreated patients and foul bathrooms. Before they could reach accreditation, Crownsville would have to embrace the techniques and therapies that doctors were implementing in other, majority-white hospitals. The APA recommended that Crownsville establish specialized departments, create formal residency and training programs, and perform medical research through ties to nearby universities.

Caught up in the pressure, staff at Crownsville desperately wanted to serve a solution to chronic problems. They saw that many of the treatments were risky, sure, but they believed trying something was better than nothing at all. And sometimes, they did produce improvements—recoveries, even.

Between 1952 and 1960, a flurry of studies involving Crownsville patients are mentioned in the records, although I was never able to find any summaries or conclusions of their findings. When I asked Paul Lurz and his friend Rob Schoeberlein, a current Maryland state archivist, why these records didn't exist, they suspected that nobody had been required to keep them, though they may have been captured as papers submitted and published in the medical journals of the era. I have not been able to find them. "The great 1950s push for research in mental hospitals involved numerous human rights violations," Paul wrote to me. At the time he arrived in the 1960s, staff were sometimes still offering patients cigarettes and candies in exchange for trying out new drugs. "P.S." he added, "I am not making any excuses for Crownsville staff. They, after all, referred the patients for the research studies."

This research ranged from studies on the intelligence of children and people with personality disorders to patients with syphilis, sickle cell, or lung cancer, and experimental procedures on people living with epilepsy, like Elsie.

It wasn't until 1962 that the Crownsville team was able to earn accreditation, but that was not because anyone had found the silver bullet for insanity. Crownsville had poked, tested, prodded, and hosed down hundreds of its patients, and yet they were hardly closer to understanding the origins of mental diseases. These contradictions and hardships were not unique to Crownsville or to Black patients. Every asylum was attempting to use what little was available during those decades. Care for the long-term mentally ill, of all races, was brutal.

In the years before anti-psychotic medication, the primary treatment available to patients at Crownsville was hydrotherapy. In bathrooms and communal showers, aides would set up deep soaking tubs. They'd take the most troublesome patients and submerge them into extreme temperatures.

A large white sheet would wrap around the tub, leaving only a small space for the patient's head to poke through. Patients would sit there, unable to move or lift their limbs, for hours or even days in icy or burning-hot water. In the archives, there are images of white nurses standing over Black men submerged below these thick, wet sheets. Employees explained that while the procedure might appear innocent, even calming, in photos, it could be incredibly uncomfortable and desta-bilizing. Often, they said, nurses would place patients in the tubs not because they believed water would cure much, but simply with the hope that it might keep a patient quiet for a while.

One of the rarer, more coercive methods of hydrotherapy was devel-oped by Benjamin Rush, a signer of the Declaration of Independence.

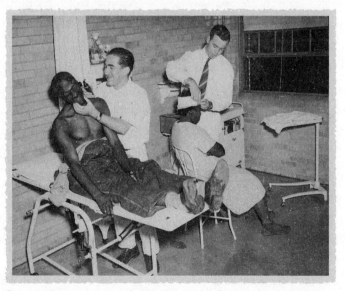

Crownsville patients treated in the hospital infirmary. A woman wears a simple dress, the man wears a workman's overalls and tattered shoes. Date unknown. From the collections of the Maryland State Archives.

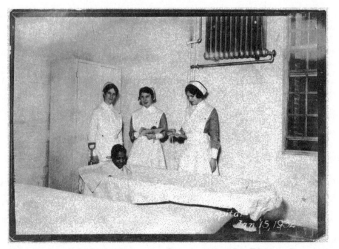

A patient receives hydrotherapy on January 15, 1932. During the treatment, a patient would be submerged in piping hot or freezing cold water for hours or days at a time. From the collections of the Maryland State Archives.

Rush designed a chair, first introduced at a hospital in Pennsylvania, that kept a patient's limbs, torso, wrists, and head all completely still. Once the patient was tied up, cold water was spilled over their head as warm water was simultaneously applied to the feet. "Its effects have been truly delightful to me," Rush stated. "It acts as a sedative to the tongue and temper as well as to the blood vessels." Rush called this sensory-deprivation and hydrotherapy chair the "Tranquilizer."

During the 1930s and 1940s, the patients seen as being the most disruptive and delusional at Crownsville and elsewhere were subjected to lobotomies. Crownsville couldn't afford to perform the notorious surgery on-site, so hospital staff would send patients who were suffering from schizophrenia or depression out to the University of Maryland for the procedure. Surgeons would take an instrument resembling an ice pick, and through a hole drilled in the patient's head or a pathway through the eye socket, they would cut and scrape away the connections between a patient's prefrontal cortex and the rest of their brain.

Proponents believed the surgery quieted a patient's overactive mind and made hospital wards more manageable. Often, they were just enjoying the sound of silence and irreversible brain damage. When Jacob Morgenstern took over as superintendent in 1947, he expressed his extreme discomfort with the practice, and the number of lobotomies quickly plummeted. They weren't nonexistent, though. A report I obtained from April 1950 noted that a Crownsville patient named William traveled to nearby Baltimore City Hospital for a lobotomy. There was no information about the procedure or his symptoms. All I could find, among other routine administrative announcements, was the news that William had died following the lobotomy. He was only thirty-three years old.

As Black employees entered the asylum, shock therapies designed to jolt and reset the brain took over. They were relatively easy to perform and didn't require much expertise. Supervisors would ask Black aides to hold the patient by their arms and legs. In some cases, employees would administer high levels of insulin to a nondiabetic person, causing them to lose consciousness, sometimes for hours, and emerge in a strange stupor. As prescription medicine became more popular among psychiatric workers, the seizure-inducing drug Metrazol was introduced for a similar effect.

But the most common method was electroshock, a procedure that Black staff members found especially painful and confusing to witness, sometimes many times a day. Employees would be asked to strap patients down and place electrodes on their skulls. A nurse would send a current surging through the patient's brain. Convulsions would come over them, sometimes so strong that patients permanently lost memories or emerged with spinal fractures. Some of the earliest Black nurses felt their patients had been coerced into an electroshock routine. It wasn't being used as a last resort; it had become as normal as taking vitamins in the morning. They worried that while these therapies were sometimes meant as genuine treatment—and some patients liked and requested them—there were teams at the hospital who seemed to leverage them as punishments.

Bearing Witness

On George Phelps's first day as a member of the Anne Arundel sheriff's department in 1951, his boss got flooded with calls. There was a Black man impersonating a police officer, they said. He had been spotted with

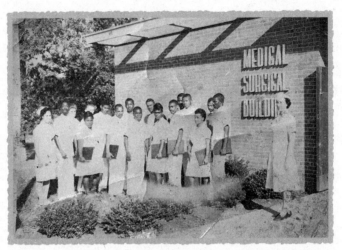

Gertrude Belt, far left, and fellow nurses line up before a shift. Super-visors would inspect their clothing, hair, and stockings before the day began. 1960s. Photo courtesy of the Belt family.

future congressman Steny Hoyer and lobbyist Bruce Bereano. Had he kidnapped them? This man was even carrying a gun.

His chief let concerned residents know that he was aware. He had hired the man.

Phelps, or as Janice Hayes-Williams calls him, Uncle George, had returned from fighting in World War II to find that most businesses and law enforcement agencies in the area were refusing to hire men like him. He tried applying to the city, the county, and the state police. The sher-iff's department finally gave him a shot.

It wasn't long before everyone knew about George. White politicians started to call on him for help, running to him when they needed to test a message with Anne Arundel's Black communities. He stood a few steps away from Martin Luther King Jr. as he delivered his "I Have a Dream" speech, standing guard as part of the security detail in Washington, D.C. George recruited a team of all-Black deputies that patrolled Carr's Beach, where Black people from all over would come to scream and shimmy at the feet of musical legends like Tina Turner and Chuck Berry, and where, after wild concerts, they'd occasionally loiter a little too late. George was funny and warm, but he was six feet, eight inches tall and had a reputa-tion for being no nonsense. Late at night, kids would split off in every direction when he'd turn the corner, and he'd come running right after them. He'd shout about how he'd drop them off at Crownsville if they didn't go home. He liked to tell kids the notorious hospital would give him twenty-five bucks in exchange for each child.

For years, he had heard rumors about the place. And more than a few times when he had come to drop someone off, it hadn't been a joke. His niece Janice Hayes-Williams can't remember the first time she heard the word Crownsville. She just knew her uncle had been there, and that it wasn't anywhere she or her friends wanted to end up.

One day, in the 1960s, George was on Crownsville's campus, walking through a parking lot that sits between the Winterode Building and the one-floor medical-surgical center. He started snooping, descending an outdoor cement staircase that led to the hospital's lab and morgue. He walked into the laboratory, where the lights were down and no one else was around. In the center was a large chemist's table with clear jars scattered about. It looked to George like each jar held a different human body part suspended in a putrid yellow-green fluid. He looked closer. One resembled a woman's womb.

"He knew the place was bad," Janice told me. "But he felt like he was in a nightmare." He stumbled backward and rushed back up the stairs before any hospital staff could spot him. George Phelps shared the story with close family and later a documentarian, but he never formally reported it to the hospital or county. Keeping autopsy specimens may seem strange but Crownsville was one of many institutions engaged in such research. Still, Janice got the sense that whatever her uncle had seen affected him deeply. He had brought his own people here, after all.

It was the same for many of the first Black people who came to Crownsville as anything other than a patient. In 1955, Marie Gough watched one morning in A Building as her white supervisor fought with a patient who had been scheduled for electroshock. The man couldn't have been more than twenty years old. He was tall, handsome, and unwilling to follow Marie's boss out of his cell.

Eventually, he slowly moved toward the door of his room. Marie thought he was caving in. Suddenly, he darted out into the hallway. As her boss chased after him, the patient raced down the narrow hallway. Before Marie could process what was happening, the young man jumped out of the nearest window to his death on the lawn below.

Administration tasked a friend of Marie's, Barbara Shank, with helping to administer electroshock in the Meyer Building. Barbara didn't question when managers told her it was part of some patient's daily routine. Four people would be assigned to hold the patient's limbs, and when possible, an extra aide would be asked to lean over the patient's middle. The doctor would then place leads on the patient's head. He'd send the first shock. The patient would writhe. The doctor would deliver another shock. The patient would convulse. Around and around they went, increasing the voltage until they reached their desired result.

Decades later, in 2022, I asked Barbara if being part of the shock team had changed her. "I was preoccupied with my job. I thought it was helping somebody," she told me. It looked as though I'd asked her a question she didn't want to linger on for too long. In the moment, when she was standing there with her team members, she explained, it didn't bother her too much. She thought it was all part of working in a big, complicated hospital. But what she witnessed stayed with her when her shifts came to an end. "It was actually a repercussion when I got home to relax and thought about what it was." The line between what was normal and professional and what was abuse wasn't always clear.

For Marie and Barbara, the stress and trauma of working on these wards took years to surface. They had arrived at Crownsville excited to care for people who looked like them, and quickly came to see they were a long way from being in charge. Black staff—and particularly Black women—were at the bottom of the hospital's social hierarchy. They didn't have the superintendent's ear and weren't setting policy. The point that went unsaid but understood was that Black people should be grateful for the chance to work at Crownsville. Keeping your head down and taking orders was part of the job.

By the time Joyce and Errol Phillip, the couple that came to Crownsville from Flint, Michigan, arrived on campus in the 1960s, the hospital's diversity had improved, but the culture and treatment were still touch and go.

Errol had grown up in the 1940s and 1950s with a father struggling with alcoholism and an older cousin who went in and out of institutionalization after having a mental breakdown and stabbing his wife. In his youth, he picked up words like "crazy" and "berserk" to describe their sicknesses—though he saw so much of it, he didn't remember knowing what depression or schizophrenia were as a child. At Crownsville, he became immersed with patients doing hours of one-on-one and group therapy. But Joyce, the manager of the Research Department, came to see Crownsville from a different vantage point.

One of the first major assignments to hit her desk in 1968 came from a wealthy benefactor who had an interest in studying the seizure drug Dilantin. Joyce's job was to help coordinate a group of patients who had previously been taking the antipsychotic Thorazine. The objective was to run an unbiased, double-blind study and find out if the seizure medicine had any effect on patients experiencing psychoses.

A double-blind study is one where neither the participants nor the researcher are aware of which treatment the participants are receiving until the conclusion. But Joyce's patients had schizophrenia, and Thorazine was a powerful drug. Often the patients taking it had visible, jittery side effects and spasms. The study didn't end up being so blind after all.

Joyce noticed something odd. Some of the patients quickly redeveloped psychoses, as she had predicted from the outset. But other patients, who had long been labeled as schizophrenic showed very negligible differences in behavior and perception after they stopped taking Thorazine. It made her question her involvement, and why and how some of the patients had come to take medication in the first place.

In the early 1970s, Errol was reading the paper one Sunday morning when he heard a commotion outside. There, passed out on the ground, was one of Crownsville's white security officers. He was surrounded by other guys on the shift, none of whom seemed to know what to do. Errol ran out in his pajamas. The officer was unresponsive, and Errol knew immediately that he was suffering a heart attack. He knelt down and began to perform CPR in the grass.

There wasn't much time to think in the moment, but Errol and this man knew each other. A few years earlier, Errol and Joyce had mentioned to a friend of theirs that they were interested in moving into a local neighborhood away from campus. That friend offered to check out a home for them. When their friend arrived, this same officer allegedly told him, "We don't want your niggers in this community."

That morning, Errol tried to save his life anyway. He died later that same day.

For employees like Barbara, Marie, and the Phillipses, there was a constant, dissonant hum. Working at Crownsville was incredibly difficult and still, somehow, the easiest decision they ever made. They resented the racist systems and segregated neighborhoods that had brought them there and brought their patients to the brink. They could hate its early history and yet thank God for the opportunity to work, to make friends, to go to nursing school, to help a few patients at a time.

Just barely past the age of eighteen, Estella and William Jones arrived at Crownsville determined to build something lasting. Bill didn't know a thing about psychiatry or medicine when he applied for a job. He was raised a country boy on the Eastern Shore in the 1940s, on land not far from where George Armwood and Matthew Williams had been lynched. He got his start in life picking beans and tomatoes. He'd help out on dairy farms and tend to cows. The work wasn't so bad but it came with no benefits, no health insurance, no path to anywhere.

Bill needed something secure. At his brother's suggestion, he took a trip to Crownsville and asked about a job. They asked him, "Well, what are you interested in?" Bill was honest. He had no clue. "What do you have open?"

The hospital needed help in every corner. Housekeeping. Groundskeeping. Laboratory workers. Bill figured the lab might work—he had always been interested in science, and he dreamed of completing his education someday. The pay wouldn't be great, they warned, but a spot in the lab came with health insurance and the promise of future raises. So Bill started as a lab assistant, taking classes at night to earn certifications. It didn't take long for him to get promoted to laboratory technician. Around that time, his future wife, Estella, came to Crownsville looking for something of her own.

She didn't need anyone's recommendation. Estella had known Crownsville since she was a child. Estella's aunt had always been a superstitious woman, but when her husband had a stroke, she became convinced someone wanted to put a hex on her family. When they'd visit, Estella would find that her aunt had poured salt all around her home, lining the base of every wall. The salt, she explained, would keep someone from "working roots" on her. Soon, salt was replaced with creosote. Her aunt would take a wide brush and paint with the dark oil distilled from coal tar. It was toxic; Estella detested the smell. But her aunt covered the walls and windows, certain it would seal her from a spell.

Estella came home one day to find that her aunt had tried to burn her grandmother's house down with her grandmother inside. Thankfully nobody was hurt, but the family couldn't go on like this. They brought her aunt to Crownsville.

Estella was nineteen when she came looking for a job as an aide. Her first memory was a smell, not a sight. An odor that seeped out of the Winterode Building. It was strange to inhale a sour, decaying scent from a beautiful, Colonial Revival–style estate.

When Estella went to get blood drawn as part of a physical for all new staff, she walked down into the Medical Surgical Building and laid eyes on her future husband. Bill, barely twenty-one, was the one drawing the samples. She liked him immediately.

During the day, Bill and his teammates would travel around to every ward, and in the afternoons Estella would come see him in the Medical Surgical Building, which the employees called Med-Surg. Bill got the chance to meet patients in every part of the campus. He would sit them down, draw their blood, and collect their urine samples. Back in the lab, the techs would run tests and update the doctors.

The laboratory gave Bill—and by extension, Estella—a different view of the hospital's potential for treatment. As women like Marie and Barbara worked draining shifts searching for physical solutions to mental troubles, Bill could see all about a patient's liver, cholesterol, and blood sugar documented on sheets of paper. He grew especially close to diabetic patients who needed him to draw their blood several times a week. Bill, like many employees before him, had started to suspect that some of his patients didn't belong at Crownsville. He could see it in their labs. They didn't have mental diseases; they had struggled with their physical health. Like him, they'd had no insurance. An infection had gone untreated. They had long been malnourished. Their bodies were failing them, and doctors were wasting time assuming it was their minds.

Bill's boss, a pathologist, noticed something in him. He asked Bill to start helping out with autopsies. Bill was leery at first. He didn't even like to watch when he got his own blood drawn. But his boss showed him the ropes.

Bill would head down to the lab early and take a patient from a freezer. He'd check to make sure he had the right body, and read the toe tags to be sure they matched the name on the autopsy schedule. He'd pull out surgical instruments and lay them out in a line. When his boss came down, he would immediately jump into the surgical process. Bill would be at his side as his boss carefully cut through patients' skin and fat.

Bill was always forced to do the dirtiest part. The first time he cut intestines and cleaned out impacted fecal matter, he almost passed out. He couldn't believe it when he helped cut a skull and held a brain in his hands. His boss would hand him organs and have him place them on a scale. Bill would fight disturbing thoughts to the back of his mind and remind himself that a country boy was here and was grateful to be learning about the human body. That didn't keep him from begging his boss to finish up before the lunch hour. He would breathe clean air and take a few minutes to recover.

Estella would try to sneak quick visits to her husband. She'd run down the stairs, peer through the small window in the Med-Surg basement door. If a patient's body was on the table, she'd turn right back around. Blood and bodily fluids weren't her thing.

Seeing what cirrhosis of the liver looked like up close changed Bill. He could see and touch what heavy medications or alcoholism had done to people he had met. It fascinated and nagged at him. It made him look differently at every sip of alcohol. He stopped taking pain-relieving medications, fearful of what their long-term use could do to his organs. Bill saw people dying younger than they should have. He removed deformed pancreases and ulcers on the stomach. "They were pushing pills," he told me. "Some places, the doctors were [pushing them] just to make sure they were calm and quiet." It felt like there was a disconnect between the enthusiasm of the doctors for the treatments they had available and the warning signs Bill could see up close.

Not every patient got an autopsy after death. Typically a patient's family agreed to one over the phone. Sometimes, when relatives didn't trust Crownsville, they'd ask for the autopsy to be done by the state-run Anatomy Board. In such cases, Med-Surg would take the body from their fridge and hand it to state employees, who'd then issue a report themselves. Bill's boss would push to do as many autopsies at Crownsville as they'd allow. That was the only way his team could understand how a person had died, and get a sense of the patients who'd been mistreated.

Estella spent years working with children and runaways. She grew close to many of her patients, and after she and Bill were married, she invited some of the ones without family to stay with them at their home. After more than three decades, Bill and Estella retired together in 1996. By that point, they were both a little disillusioned. They loved their teams and the life they had built together. Crownsville had put their kids through college and helped their family afford land in Anne Arundel. But budgets were slashed year after year. Patients were being sent out onto the streets to return to the "community," although it seemed there was no plan for their continuing care. Bill had seen countless bodies—and Estella had worked with generations of kids, adults, and families. Estella knew it was time to go when they started to dread waking up in the morning.

As integration continued, Crownsville slowly shed the plantation structure. Employees worked hard so that a reputation for therapy and professionalism might solidify in its place. After seeing conditions of obvious cruelty from the outside, they were proud that they worked at an institution that was now home to some of the most diverse and open-minded people in the medical field.

Some power dynamics proved to be intractable, however. Diversity and representation helped, but they couldn't erase the basic facts of their chosen profession. For all the tests, shocks, and surgeries performed, patients could still fall through the cracks and they were still no closer to a cure.

Deborah and Her Sister

Henrietta visited Elsie religiously for a couple of years, even with a handful of young children at home and doctor's appointments and treatments that she wished to keep secret. For some time, Henrietta had been suffering through severe abdominal pain and vaginal bleeding. She felt like there was a knot in her stomach that wouldn't go away.

Henrietta underwent a series of procedures and treatments for what was determined to be cervical cancer. During a biopsy, her cells were harvested for testing. Those cells would go on to save an unimaginable number of lives, but they wouldn't save hers. Her visits to Elsie came to an end as the cancer metastasized throughout her body. Henrietta died in October 1951 at the age of thirty-one.

According to Rebecca Skloot, the last time Henrietta saw Elsie, she was seated outside in one of the patient courtyards behind a barbed wire fence. Henrietta peered through the wiring and made eye contact with her daughter. Elsie jumped and ran to her mom. For a moment, she stood there staring. "She look like she doin' better," Henrietta said to a family friend, almost as though she was trying to convince herself it would be okay—as though she knew it was the last day she'd have with her child. "Yeah, Elsie look nice and clean and everything."

When her mother was laid to rest, people came for days to see her body in the old home-house. Nobody, it seemed, thought to bring Elsie.

Years went by before Elsie's younger sister, Deborah, learned the truth. When she found out what doctors had done to her mother, and how taxing it was to get institutions like Johns Hopkins to tell her the truth, she began to worry about what might have been done to Elsie.

Deborah called Crownsville's administration to demand access to her sister's records. They claimed that almost every document from before 1955 had been destroyed. Conveniently, that was the year Elsie died at the asylum. It didn't sit right with Deborah's spirit. She broke out in hives and struggled to catch her breath. When she checked in to see her doctor, he told her she had almost had a stroke.

Rebecca Skloot and Deborah Lacks made a trip to Crownsville. Deborah tucked an old photo of Elsie into her purse before the long drive, along with Elsie's birth certificate and proof of power of attorney.

The two women came across Paul Lurz. Paul was then serving as Crownsville's director of performance and improvement. Already he had a reputation as an unofficial historian who had access to decades of records. As he pulled out files, he warned them: "Sometimes learning can be just as painful as not knowing."

Paul disappeared into a closet. When he emerged, he was carrying a series of old autopsy reports, blanketed with stains and dust. Paul and Deborah quickly found the report bearing Elsie's name. In her file was a photograph. In it, Elsie's wide chestnut eyes, which once rested beautifully beneath her curls, were nearly swollen shut and bulging from her head. The curls that Henrietta had so adored were matted and frizzy; her lips were dry, dark, and twice their former size. Two large, white, manicured hands gripped Elsie's once beautiful neck, twisting her gaze to the left and holding her in place. It appeared Deborah's sister was screaming.

Records from 1955, the year that Elsie died—and the year Marie Gough got her start at Crownsville, two years before Gertrude Belt was hired—indicate that doctors at Crownsville performed two studies on people with epilepsy that year. One titled "Use of Deep Temporal Leads in the Study of Psychomotor Epilepsy" suggested that doctors had tested new or more aggressive forms of shock to patients' brains. Another from that same year was titled "Pneumoencephalographic and Skull and X-ray Studies in 100 Epileptics." There were only about a hundred people with epilepsy at the hospital at the time, meaning there was almost no doubt Elsie, who had no ability to communicate or to consent, had been forced to take part.

This was an unusually brutal treatment, one that none of the employees of color that I've spoken to had experienced or seen. Pneumoencephalography required doctors to drill into a patient's skull to drain out the fluid that surrounds each and every one of our brains. Air or helium would be pumped into the skull, allowing physicians to produce sharp X-rays of a person's brain. The process was as painful as it sounds and had the potential to permanently disfigure. It could take months for a person to restore their brain fluid to normal levels. In the meantime, they would suffer headaches, seizures, and fits of vomiting. I was able to obtain Elsie's death certificate, but never her autopsy report. People who've seen it say the records indicate that in the last six months of her life, Elsie forcibly vomited almost daily, frequently coughing up dark brown clotted blood.

Deborah Lacks had every right to be outraged. Discussions of informed consent may not have been as rigorously regulated as they are today, but they have been part of the medical field since the turn of the twentieth century. Crownsville had a duty to its patients and to their families. Winterode may have been long gone by the time Elsie died, but his legacy was lingering. The imagery of a white staffer gripping Elsie's neck and forcing her into submission mirrored many of the hospital's earliest photographs. In an attempt to appear professional and capable of advanced study, Crownsville staff had actually entrenched old habits under a clinical cover.

That day in Paul's office, he, Deborah, and Rebecca stood together, often in silent shock. Deborah pulled out the old, beautiful photo she had brought with her. She placed it next to the other, almost unrecognizable version of her big sister. Paul and Rebecca watched as Deborah traced her fingers along Elsie's bruised face. She whispered, "She looks like she needs her sister."

CHAPTER 13

Nurse Faye and Sonia King

FAYE BELT WAS BREATHING HEAVILY. HER BRAIN WENT ON AUTOPI-lot as she hightailed it across Crownsville's back lawns. She whizzed past the old barns and beyond the Campanella recreation building. She was approaching the woods near Cottage 13, closing in on a young man twenty feet in front of her. He was a patient, and she knew him well—he worked with her mom, Gertrude. When all the other patients were pre-occupied with a game and nobody was looking, the young man had made a break for it. It was a valiant effort, but in another universe, Faye Belt was probably a high jumper or professional sprinter. She had let him have a thirty-second head start, and laughed to herself as he made his way toward a stream. Neither of them knew how to swim. She leapt on him from behind and tackled him to the ground. "Goddamn," he chuckled. "I heard about you."

One of the other aides followed behind Faye a few minutes later. They were always grateful that the Belt kids were so fast. Whenever Faye caught up to a patient, she'd wait with them, cracking jokes about how they got caught by a teenager. *Now, why would you sprint toward the water? When you could've run toward the cornfields and the main road?*

Then Faye would lie down in the grass. She'd tug at the weeds and look up at the clouds gliding over her head. In those days, Crownsville still smelled of pigs, cows, and manure. She'd breathe it all in and recover from her run.

Faye understood that this was not how most junior high schoolers spent their afternoons after school in the 1960s. But if you asked her, she'd say it was better that she catch you than the Anne Arundel police or God knows what back in those woods. For Faye, being asked if she found growing up inside an asylum strange is sort of like asking a person if they'd paid much attention to their breathing. That was life, and she wasn't going to spend too much time dwelling on it.

And in fact, the asylum was not the strangest and most alienating place in Faye's adolescence. By the time she was a student at Arundel Senior High, Faye had become uncomfortably aware of racial tensions simmering in Annapolis. She was one of a tight pack of Black classmates who would read and watch reports about the Civil Rights Movement with family but often avoided discussing that same topic with the rest of their school. Her city, with its narrow streets and shining waterfront, was always so good at glossing over the anger and humiliation just below its surface. At least at Crownsville, everyone she spent time with was of a similar lived experience. They were honest—maybe too honest—about what they were going through. Faye learned all her first curse words from the patients and overworked nurses. They'd throw words around she'd never heard before, and she'd try to copy them. One afternoon a group of staffers hollered and clapped when they heard Gertrude's teenage daughter shout, "What the fuck?"

School was not always so easy. In 1970, when Faye was a junior, she decided to try out for the Arundel High cheerleading squad. Gertrude left the hospital and came down to the school gym to watch her daughter's audition routine through a window. She had no doubt Faye would make the team. It wasn't just patients at Crownsville who'd heard about how athletic she was. Gertrude remembered staring at a girl with red hair who walked out on the floor right before Faye, and how it looked like she was struggling with her splits and jumps. By the time Faye stepped forward, Gertrude beamed with pride as her daughter landed all her flips and splits.

She was shocked the next day when Faye came home bawling. The redhead had made the team. Faye hadn't. Gertrude marched right back to the school and asked to meet the principal.

The principal asked her a rhetorical question. "What's best for the community?"

Gertrude seethed. "What do you mean what's best for the community?" The next day Faye joined the rest of the cheerleaders.

The following year, in the twelfth grade, Faye rode to school at the front of an Arundel High bus labeled number 158. It made its usual stop at the Junior High, turned around a bend, and curved up a small hill toward the upperclassmen's building. Faye sat up straight. She squinted. There by the entrance doors to her high school in white, sloppy paint were the words "Niggers Go Home."

Faye started yelling and asking who did it. The driver, an older woman the kids called Mrs. Pippen, pulled the bus around and shouted at Faye to behave. Faye leapt off and linked arms with a few girlfriends. She stood on top of a low brick wall outside the school, shouting to her classmates, *Look at this!* She gathered up every Black student she could find. They marched into the high school assembly hall and stood together at the edge of the stage. None of them really knew how to hold a protest. They put up their fists, like they'd seen their favorite Black athletes and activists do. They started to chant, "We're not leaving! We're not leaving!" Teachers rushed in, demanding that all of them head back to class or risk punishment. Faye balked. "You can call my mom," she warned. "Try it." By lunchtime, the administration had washed those words away. Faye went back to class.

So, when Faye would get home to Crownsville there was a wave of relief. She'd fly off the school bus and stroll into the employee cafeteria. She'd say hi to her mom's friends as she helped herself to hamburgers and vanilla soft serve from a machine. Someone gave her her own copy of staff keys for the canteen, library, and recreation room. She could open the library and the recreation room and pick out snacks and toys for herself and the other employees' kids and patients they hung out with. She and her siblings, Frederica and Frederick, would walk across

Crownsville Road and trudge up the winding driveway to the superintendent's home. They'd push each other in his pool and chase each other
around until he got home from the office or asked them to leave. At
Crownsville, all the employees and all the patients knew or had heard of
the Belt kids. She felt safer there than almost anywhere else.

Faye and her siblings planned football and softball tournaments when
the weather was good, and they refused to go easy on anybody, including
the patients. On Thursdays, the Belts would attend movie night in the
Grove, a favorite grassy hangout sandwiched between the HY Building
and a baseball field. Staff would hang a movie screen out there on the
days it didn't rain. In July, Faye would talk up the annual Family Day
parade to any patient who would listen. The Crownsville administration would spend a little money on small floats and decorations, and cars
would go driving down the road that cut in front of the Meyer Building. It looked like their own Independence Day parade. Patients would
invite their relatives to travel in from all over. They'd lay out blankets
and they'd sit out on the lawn for hours. Employees would blast music
from the Campanella building, and the hospital cooks would bring hot
finger foods out on trucks. Even the sickest patients were allowed outside on Family Day. Faye and other employees' kids walked around the
lawn, handing out balloons and wildflowers. Her mom's friend and colleague, Dorothea McCullers, would mend and prepare the patients' best
clothes. For the patients who didn't have anyone to visit, the Belt kids
would stand in. Faye could make conversation with a brick wall.

Nobody was surprised when Faye's afternoons playing softball turned
into college summers spent volunteering at the hospital. They hardly noticed
when she turned those stints into her first full-time job as an aide. When
Faye passed her Board exam, a village showed up to scream and shout at her
commencement ceremony. On August 19, 1977, at twenty-four years old,
Faye walked across a stage at the Maryland Vocational Rehabilitation Center
wearing bright white clinic shoes and a white dress with buttons all down
the front. She received her practical nursing degree from the Department of
Health and Mental Hygiene. She made a show of it, jumping up and down
and taking a bow as she held onto her certificate.

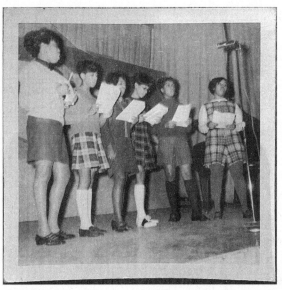

Faye Belt, third from the right, performs with other children during a hospital talent show. Late 1960s. Photo courtesy of the Belt family.

Faye got a call one afternoon in January 1979. A new patient in the Meyer Building wished to see her. When this person arrived, staff had to pry her out of her family's car. She didn't want to walk and wouldn't move toward the admission doors. A nurse had tried to serve her medication. The patient, they claimed, was paranoid and had slapped the small white cup of meds out of the nurse's hands. Staff forced her into a seclusion cell. For twenty-four hours, even the patient's family hadn't been able to see her.

It was Sonia King. A friend and one of the younger sisters of Faye's classmate Herbie from Arundel High. The last time Faye and Sonia had seen each other was at a Sunday service with extended family and friends at Macedonia United Methodist Church in Odenton. Sonia had always been quieter and less self-assured than the Belt kids, carefully considering her words before she spoke, but she was always well liked. She was the daughter of Odessa and Herbert King, a Korean War veteran who had moved his family from Fort Knox, Kentucky, to Fort Meade, Maryland. Faye and Sonia had bonded over a mutual obsession with sports and competition. Sonia was a scholar-athlete, recruited for basketball by one of the oldest historically Black colleges and universities in the country, Lincoln University. She arrived at Crownsville at just twenty years old.

Faye rushed to find her. She got permission from the nurse on duty to take Sonia out for a private walk. She squeezed Sonia in tight. "What happened? What's going on with the family?"

Sonia started to explain. That New Year's Eve, the King family drove to a friend's house party in Washington, D.C. The entire extended family sat down around a large living room, eating, drinking, and playing a game of Family Feud. When one of her siblings started reading prompts off a playing card, Sonia would reply with off-the-wall answers. Her parents and brother started to sense something was off. "Come on, Son, please stop playing," they said, laughing.

Sonia's littlest sister started to cry out for a toy, her "doll-baby," that she had left behind in the family car. Sonia, overcome by anxiety and desperate for fresh air, offered to go grab it. Her sister handed her the car keys. Sonia asked her what kind of car the family had. They stared back at her funny. She'd been in it a million times before. "Sonia, stop it. Please cut this out."

Sonia stepped out into the night. She doesn't remember what she was doing, why it took her so long to figure out how to get into the car. Her brother Perry followed behind to see what was going on. He said, "Girl, just give me the keys." Sonia started to scream. "No, Perry! Don't go! They're going to shoot you! They're going to kill you!"

Perry ran back inside. The party was over. The family rushed Sonia to the Walter Reed Army Medical Center, where doctors asked her a series of reality and orientation questions. *Who's the president? What's the date?*

The doctors told Sonia that she was depressed and on the verge of having a nervous breakdown. She needed to be hospitalized. But Walter Reed had no rooms. The next day, her parents took her to an emergency room in Baltimore. She was becoming more and more paranoid. She wouldn't answer the phone. She didn't trust the staff and wouldn't take any of their medicine. They told her that if she didn't start to cooperate, they were going to send her somewhere that would force her to.

That's how Sonia came to Crownsville. Even today, she doesn't understand why nurses wanted to force medicine into her so quickly without asking her what she had been going through. She was afraid. "She should have got my medical record," Sonia said of the first nurse she encountered there. "She should have had some medical history."

If the nurse had asked, Sonia would have told her about how this was the worst year of her life. She had entered her sophomore year at Lincoln University, eager to make friends. She was an athlete, but she was struggling to find her place in the school. Sonia yearned to feel like a part of something and decided to rush Zeta Phi Beta with eleven other young women. Because she was one of the quietest women on the line, the members sized her up and forced her into the role of line president. This meant that members expected Sonia to lead the other pledges in every assignment or errand. At one point, Sonia saw a member punch a pledge so hard her teeth fell out. She didn't know how to handle it. Nobody listened to her or respected her. She felt like she was drowning in tasks and failing to make the connections she had imagined.

Lincoln University was out in the middle of nowhere near Pennsylvania's Ku Klux Klan territory. The members would take Sonia and the other girls and leave them out on back roads in the middle of the night. The last thing Sonia could remember hearing a member say was, "Get back to campus the best you know how." She would quietly pray to the sky. She knew this wasn't personal. It had been done before to all who'd pledged. But there was a breaking point.

She dropped line. Sonia became depressed and isolated herself from everyone. She would go to class, eat her meals, and hide in her room for the rest of the day. Her family would try to call. She would rush them off the phone and tell them she was doing fine.

When she came home for the Christmas holidays she started to take walks alone in Odenton, Maryland, late in the night. Her sister Darnetta started to worry and asked Sonia to sleep on her bedroom floor. Darnetta wouldn't rest until she had seen Sonia lying there. They all knew Sonia was lonely at school, but they couldn't understand how fragile she'd become.

During the holiday period that same year, a male friend in the neighborhood had asked Sonia to come by and help him with something. She
said yes. But when she got there, it became clear he had something else in
mind. He raped her.

Sonia kept saying no, over and over. She kicked and fought as hard as
she could. But she was completely overpowered by the boy, a wrestler and
young recruit in the army. Afterward, Sonia didn't tell a soul. But when
she found out she was pregnant and had contracted a sexually transmitted
disease, Sonia had to tell her mom and sister, although she refused to tell
her brothers and especially her dad. "He would've been in jail for killing
the guy," she figured.

Her brother had always been close to her. He sensed this boy had done
something and offered to help Sonia get back at him. When her mom got
wind of his plans, she told him no. God would take care of the boy. The
women of the family quietly arranged for Sonia to get an abortion.

By New Year's, Sonia felt profoundly alone and hollow. She couldn't
process the intensity of rejection from women on her college campus, and
back at home, a boy had taken what was left of her sense of self. "I had
been raped and just didn't feel good enough," she explained to me. "The
whole 'damaged goods' thing. I didn't think anybody would want me." It
would be years before Sonia would start to believe she was worthy again.

Four to five days a week, Faye would finish up her shift and come meet
Sonia. Sonia was relieved to see the face of someone who understood her,
someone who, in her mind, knew the past version of her that was whole.

Faye would take Sonia's hand or they'd link arms and squeeze each
other as they looked out on Crownsville's grounds. Sonia was still refusing to swallow medicine on her own, but a nurse had given her a shot of
something by force. Sonia remembers looking across the farmland and
realizing that the medication was working. She was becoming less paranoid and she could feel in her bloodstream how the medication made her
feel like she was flying at a mile a minute. Faye did her best to make light
of it all. She would joke about their families and make it her goal to hear
Sonia laugh.

Faye would take Sonia down to the Grove, the grassy hangout where patients and employees would picnic and relax when the weather was good. Faye would sit down in the grass and spend most of the time they had together listening. Sonia needed a lot of love. She was finding it hard to open up to the social workers and doctors, but easier to confide in Faye.

Faye remembered hearing the story of Sonia's rape. She remembered how her friend would cling to her as she cried, how her lips would tremble as she talked. Faye chose her words very carefully. She wanted Sonia to know she was there and that she understood, but she knew from her own experience with an assault that what Sonia needed was to slowly rebuild her trust and faith in others. Not listen to Faye preach or recount her own traumas.

Sonia didn't like it on the ward with other patients. It was overcrowded. The beds were all crammed together, and each one had its own tiny closet container—all that a patient had to keep their worldly possessions. It looked to her like many of the patients weren't getting attention from anyone. Some of the patients would steal her clothes when she wasn't looking. One of the boys stole her Arundel High School ring and never gave it back.

Faye and other nurses did what they could to look out for her. They pulled strings to move her to a private bedroom and get her her own lock on the door. Faye remembers calling Sonia's parents and promising them she would have their back. Sonia's mom would come drop off home-cooked meals and fresh clothing. Almost every day, Sonia's mom, Odessa, would call Cottage 16 and ask to speak to Faye. She wanted the assurance that someone who cared had seen her daughter. Sonia didn't know it at the time, but she was on a "one-to-one plan," a suicide prevention plan requiring that at least one staff member always be near her.

Sonia was often bored, and she could tell that the nurses were overworked—so she offered to help them serve food to patients on her floor who needed some assistance. She volunteered to teach other patients basketball and would take groups of patients to the Crownsville gym for games. In exchange for her help, nurses gave her special privileges. They'd always let her take the last shower at night so she could have the bathroom all to herself.

A nurse named Geraldine Cully became a second mother to Sonia. She would come find her and remind her that there was something special about her. She wouldn't be in Crownsville long, Geraldine promised. The King family's pastor and the friends that had hosted Sonia on New Year's Eve came to visit her often, determined to keep her connected to life outside of the hospital. She was surrounded by family. Sonia came to trust that she could start over again. This would not be the end of her story.

Crownsville was still far from perfect; in fact, life as a patient was often heartbreaking and bizarre. What made the difference to Sonia was that she was being cared for by people who knew her and loved her and who never doubted that she had a future. She credits the Black women who wrapped their arms around her as having saved her life.

Three months later, Sonia's family came to take her home. The doctors and nurses assured the King family that they would support her care from afar, and Sonia would remain on medication as she slowly readjusted to school and daily life. Faye remembers standing in the hallway, cheering as she watched Sonia walk out of the Meyer Building's doors for the last time. She promised Sonia they would always be connected. They still are.

PART FOUR

Black Power and Pathology

1960–1980

1960: **2,038 Patients**
1980: **550 Patients**

CHAPTER 14

Screaming at the Sky

But Moses said to the people, "Do not fear! Stand by and see the salvation of the LORD which He will accomplish for you today; for the Egyptians whom you have seen today, you will never see them again forever. The LORD will fight for you while you keep silent."

—Exodus 14:13, New American Standard Bible

WE ARE OFTEN TAUGHT THAT THE GREAT MIGRATION WAS A massive migratory march brought about by a simple realization. We learned that in the early 1900s, Black families caught wind of better jobs, security, and social opportunities that would be available to them if only they could save enough money for a train ticket, pack up their belongings, and find their way to more enlightened cities like Detroit, New York, and Chicago. I remember reading about the factories and the foundries where they sought jobs, the neighborhoods and new schools that they brought to life. I heard stories about travelers dropping to their knees as they crossed the border from the South to the North, thanking God for delivering them out of the South just as Moses had delivered the Israelites out of Egypt. In my mind I saw pictures of couples and friends traveling together through the decades, climbing with their kids onto trains, and eagerly abandoning the hostile South and the oppressively hot agricultural fields. Poverty and racism were the motivating factors, but the masses were making a clear choice. It was a straightforward story, and in so many ways it felt like a triumphant one.

As I got a little older, though, I found out from family—not from my schoolteachers—that many never wanted to leave at all. That they often had less than twenty-four hours to plan their departure, and the stakes were not this-job-or-that-job; they were sometimes life or death. For these families, this Great Migration was not a careful and calculated choice—it was terrorism. It was a sudden expulsion. And as much as it had the power to lift Black families up, the journey north had the power to break them down.

Everyone describes my great-grandfather Clarence Joseph Washington as kind, musically talented, and a little awkward. He was born on September 21, 1900, in St. Petersburg, Florida, when his mom, Sophia, was just sixteen years old. Nobody knows what happened to Clarence's father—I've never heard his name—but Sophia married a nineteen-year-old man named Albert Brunson, and he took Clarence in as his stepson. Little is known about Clarence's early years. But through oral history and sparse recordkeeping, I know that Clarence left Florida as a teen to attend the historically Black college Morris Brown in Georgia. It was there that he met my future great-grandmother Ethel Valeria Washington.

Clarence and Ethel Valeria made the Great Migration in the 1940s. They left the South not by choice but by force.

On campus, Clarence was well known as the concertmaster of the college orchestra and a brilliant violinist. My living relatives have few memories of Clarence, but the one thing that always surfaces is the sound of his violin. His old instrument was the one piece of him that people held on to. They kept it in my father's childhood home in Detroit long after they had given up on him, and long after he had passed away.

The couple were from two different worlds. Clarence came from humble beginnings on the Florida coast. Ethel Valeria was the polished daughter of a successful Black doctor, from a family that was regularly featured in publications like the 1917 Georgia edition of *History of the American Negro and His Institutions* and the 1941 edition of a manual called *Who's Who in Colored America*. Her father, Joshua Sloan Williams Sr., had become one of the first Black physicians to practice in Eatonton and Macon, Georgia, in 1911. He had traveled to Canada, seen every region of the United States as a Pullman porter serving railroad passengers in sleeping cars, and then enjoyed a booming business serving Black patients. He built his practice in Georgia to fill a particular gap, prioritizing a patient population that depended on him for high-quality healthcare they could not get from white physicians—who often refused to see them or made them wait in segregated back rooms, where they would always be languishing, last in line behind any white patient who came through the door.

Not long after Clarence and Ethel Valeria graduated from college, Joshua Sloan decided that his daughter and her husband should live closer to him. Clarence was struggling to make it as a musician. When that didn't pay the bills, he struggled trying to sell life insurance. They moved into Joshua Sloan's home on Monroe Street in Macon, where my grandmother, Ethel's namesake, was born in 1929.

It was the Great Depression, and the racial politics of the time were frightening and unstable. In Georgia, the local agricultural economy had been buckling from a drought, technological change, low cotton prices, and an insect—the boll weevil—destroying existing crops. But the global financial crash pushed families to the breaking point, and Georgians of all backgrounds were going door-to-door, begging neighbors for food, and giving up basic necessities like clothing and shoes. In these conditions, Black families weren't expected to thrive. They were famously the first to be fired and the last to be hired when jobs became available again. Many fled north as a means of survival. But at first, Joshua's medical practice insulated my entire family from the chaos. My grandmother would listen intently whenever her parents answered a knock at the door. She would eavesdrop as her father, Clarence, spoke with white men who came by every week, hat in hand, to beg *her* family for food.

Being Black and comfortable made them visible, and being visible put them in danger. Not only did the family keep their home and business and send one kid or cousin off to college and medical school after another, they also became deeply involved in the church and local politics, eventually helping to establish the Macon chapter of the NAACP. They started to notice that local white reporters would include their names in almost any piece about Black advancements in Georgia. In particular, Joshua Sloan and his son Josh Jr. would show up repeatedly in the news, even if they were only loosely connected to the featured events. This was not taken as a compliment. To them, it was a threat. It felt as though the media wanted white Georgians to know exactly who they were, and where they lived, and what they did. Unease set in among the Joshuas, Ethel Valeria, and Clarence. Clarence and Ethel Valeria sent their daughter—my grandmother—to live with her aunt and uncle in Washington, D.C.

Then came the phone calls at all hours of the night. "You have twenty-four hours to leave," they'd whisper. "Niggers, we're going to kill you."

The beginning of the end came when Josh Jr. became president of the Macon NAACP. The attorney general of Georgia, a staunch opponent of integration named Eugene Cook, announced he would revoke the license of any teacher associated with the National Association for the Advancement of Colored People. Josh Jr. felt compelled to fight.

In a speech titled "The Ugly Truth About the NAACP," Eugene Cook told an association of police officers in Atlanta that the racial aims of the Communist Party of the United States and those of the NAACP were virtually identical. He laid out their overlapping goals:

"Full racial equality.

"Abolition of all laws which result in segregation of negroes.

"Abolition of all laws forbidding intermarriage of persons of different races.

"Abolition of all laws and public administration measures which prohibit, or in practice prevent, negro children from attending general public schools or universities.

"Full and equal admittance of negroes to all waiting rooms, restaurants, hotels and theaters."

The top law enforcement official of the state had compiled what he believed to be proof of Black collaboration with the Communist Party and the subversive, anti-American nature of the NAACP—and by association, our family. He concluded that they "pose a serious threat to the peace, tranquility, government, and way of life of our State."

Josh Jr. took Cook to court and beat him. The phone calls just got worse.

Soon it became too much to bear. The family story goes that one day, Clarence saw yet another news story that mentioned the family, and something snapped. The entire family believed the Ku Klux Klan had long been eyeing them, but Clarence now sensed that something was about to happen. He bought a pair of train tickets and took off with his son CJ—my grandmother's older brother—for Detroit, a city they had never seen, with a promise to send for his wife, Ethel Valeria, and the rest of the kids.

Clarence and CJ arrived in Detroit with nothing. No job, no close contacts, nowhere to sleep. For weeks, Clarence and seventeen-year-old CJ slept outside on benches on Belle Isle, an island in the Detroit River. In a matter of hours, they went from being part of one of the most prominent families in Macon to waking up every morning and going down to a bus station to bathe and dress in the public bathroom.

Eventually, Clarence found a job as a foreman for Great Lakes Steel, and Joshua Sloan Sr. bought him and Ethel Valeria a home on the East Side of Detroit. Josh Jr. gave up on Georgia and joined them, too. The North was foreign and cold, and Clarence's demeanor shifted with it. While much of Ethel's family had traveled the country and experienced its climates, Clarence had never lived with anything but the humid summers and timid winters of Florida and Georgia. Everyone was anxious about starting anew, but Clarence looked like he was in a constant state of shock. He wouldn't talk and couldn't relax. He seemed to be in a trance, at peace only in quiet moments when he could sit and play his violin at home, or when he'd go for long, wandering walks after shifts at the steel mill.

His wife didn't know how to handle it. Truth be told, Ethel Valeria resented his new blue-collar job, too. Despite losing everything they had shared in Macon, the family was trying to present a united and harmonious front in Detroit. Clarence's bitterness was an inconvenience, and she was angry that he made no attempt to keep up appearances.

We don't know much about what it was like for Clarence working at a steel plant. But the work of historians offers some clues. At the end of the nineteenth century, steel mills often used formerly enslaved people as strikebreakers against white union employees—a move that not only undermined the union's bargaining efforts but also intentionally fostered racial animus and suspicion. By 1901, U.S. Steel became the largest corporation in the world through a merger overseen by infamous banker J. P. Morgan, and this newly formed megacorporation controlled everything in its industry from start to finish—from the mines and raw materials to processes and steel products. By the mid-1900s, Black American workers, many of them fleeing the South to cities like Detroit and Pittsburgh, played a crucial role in the operation of steel mills around the country, but were consistently pushed into the most dangerous and least desirable jobs. Black employees were often assigned to the furnaces, where they were provided with limited safety equipment and clothing. Horrible burns and life-altering accidents were routine. The sounds were loud and all-consuming—like the hum and crunch of machinery and the whip and crack of dangerous flames. According to worker testimony and a national lawsuit, Black steelworkers faced constant harassment and discrimination from both their bosses and the unions that were supposed to represent them. In one scene in a documentary titled *Struggles in Steel: A Story of African-American Steelworkers*, a Black steelworker recounts how a new white man would arrive at the foundry and Black employees would be asked to train him. "In two weeks—he was your boss."

One night at the foundry, Clarence couldn't work or focus. He began to wail and cry out incoherently on his line, frightening all of the men working at his side. He walked out of his job at Great Lakes Steel and wandered along the highway for hours. When it got late and nobody had seen or heard from him, my grandmother's sister, Alma, went out driving and searched desperately for him. She found Clarence shaking and chattering alone on the road, screaming to someone in the sky.

For the rest of his life, Clarence cycled in and out of local emergency centers and the Eloise Asylum in Westland, Michigan. His breakdown created a fault line in our family. There was the before and the after. There were times of calm and times of crisis. There were those who maintained a relationship with him, and those who would barely speak of him.

One day in the early 1960s, Clarence came to see his daughter, my grandmother, Ethel, in the home my father grew up in on Detroit's Oakman Boulevard. This is the same home where years later, Cousin Maynard would begin to show signs of a paranoid spiral. My grandmother, the one Clarence sent away from Georgia so young, had married a lawyer and started her family. She was committed to the story that she came from greatness in Macon, but less forthcoming about how her family landed in Detroit.

Clarence came by, the story goes, hoping to ask Ethel why she never visited him at the hospital, why she seemed embarrassed to bring him around his grandchildren, why she hosted dinners and went to parties in the city as though her father's house wasn't just a few miles to the east.

But when the door swung open, none of the words came out. All Clarence did was lunge at his daughter in a rage. And almost as though she had seen the confrontation coming, my grandmother ducked under Clarence's arms, sprinted out of her own house, and ran down the street away from her father.

My grandmother's Aunt Betty came to check in on her later that evening. Betty was married to Josh Jr., who had himself suffered emotionally in the years following legal battles and work with the NAACP in

Georgia. She had long observed this family that she joined, confused by their unwillingness to simply talk about what had happened. Why did everyone want to act and dress like they hadn't just lost everything? Why was nobody driving to Eloise Asylum to visit Clarence—whose paranoia and instincts might actually be the only reason they were all still alive? Why insist that Detroit was your American Dream when it was the escape from a nightmare?

She saw so much anger toward Clarence. The family was embarrassed, intent on leaving him out as the crazy one because he was honest about how scared and lost he was. All the while, the rest of them were playing one big game of make-believe. One afternoon, about sixty years ago, she tried to ask Ethel the same questions that were on Clarence's spirit. And when I called her in the fall of 2022, those very same questions were still frustrating my ninety-one-year-old great-aunt, who had outlived them all.

Betty says she told my grandmother that she had one of two choices to make. She could try to understand her father's affliction and come to terms with all of the loss and the hurt. Or she would need to go buy better tennis shoes to outrun him.

My grandmother chose to keep running.

CHAPTER 15

The Curious Case of the Elkton Three

J UANITA NELSON DROVE WHILE HER LIFE PARTNER, WALLY, SAT SHOT-
gun. The two always looked like they had been made for each other,
their wide smiles often wrinkling the corners of their eyes in unison.
Juanita wore her hair relaxed and pinned back. Often Wally was a little
looser—a few buttons undone on his shirt and a few days behind in his
shaving. In the back seat, their roommate and best friend, Eroseanna,
or Rose, looked out of the window with a scarf on her head, staring out
at the dusty four-lane highway called Route 40. The trio were heading
home from a visit to Washington, D.C., where they had gone to check on
a friend who was being held in a psychiatric ward. That friend had been
arrested for protesting taxes and war—something this group of friends
had protested together many times before. They were exhausted, doing
their best to make their way back to the Powelton Village neighborhood
of Philadelphia.

The road they were on was not just any small-town throughway.
And some small part of Juanita, Wally, and Rose knew that they might
not make it home that night at all. As they passed all the trees thin-
ning out for the start of the fall, and read the names of all the roadside
greasy-spoon food spots, a certain electricity moved between them. They
arrived in Elkton, Maryland.

Today, the Mason-Dixon Line exists primarily in our national imagination as a symbol of all that has historically and culturally separated the North from Confederate Dixie. But in the early 1960s, it was very real. One could see and feel a shift as they passed from Pennsylvania or Delaware into the state of Maryland. Though Route 40 looked unremarkable, it was one of the nation's busiest highways and, for a time, a central artery that controlled passage from North to South. Black Americans and their families couldn't travel through this artery carelessly; they had to know what these lines—physical and imaginary—meant. In 1961, entering Maryland meant no more meals or stops to use the restroom. Black people were openly and regularly denied service at restaurants, stores, and hotels once over the border.

Route 40 was home to dozens of segregated restaurants, the kind that proudly hung "Whites Only" signs out front. Even African diplomats, traveling through Maryland for business with our State Department, were not able to stop for coffee. Stokely Carmichael, a beloved Black Power leader and chair of the Student Nonviolent Coordinating Committee, once spoke about the unique humiliations of traveling along Route 40 as a college student. "I developed a deep hatred—one shared by many—for Route 40," he wrote in his book *Ready for Revolution*. Soon, local activists saw the road as an opportunity for a special kind of nonviolent disobedience. They'd enter a business or a public place and remain seated until forcibly evicted, in protest of the establishment's racist, segregationist policies. These sit-ins, which began in South Carolina in 1960, helped integrate countless local businesses across more than twenty states.

An organization called the Congress of Racial Equality (CORE) would distribute brochures, making clear which restaurants served all travelers and which were dangerous. It was a *Green Book* of sorts. They urged their followers and made signs: "Help Complete the Job. End Racial Discrimination Along US 40."

Juanita, Wally, and Rose would do their part.

The trio spotted the Bar-H Chuck House, a small diner they had never seen before, with a bright green roof and striped trim above the windows, advertising the basics like sandwiches and homemade ice cream. Juanita pulled the car into the parking lot, with Route 40 stretching out behind them. All she remembered thinking was that this kind of truck stop would give a good portion of food and not be all that expensive. Years later she still questioned it. "I don't know why we didn't think about it."

Many times before, these three had found themselves at the precipice. Most of their lives and much of their friendship had been built around finding the heart to cross a line or take a leap of faith. Wally, in particular, was usually calm and peaceful, someone who cared about people's internal struggles and could be blissfully unaware of the danger his own skin could put them in. "He saw the color in another person's eyes, and the sparkle in the other person's eyes, and he looked right on through and saw what was inside, and what happened to be the wrapping just didn't make any difference to Wally," a friend once recalled.

Juanita and Wally had fallen in love when Juanita was a reporter and Wally was an inmate at the Cuyahoga County Jail. Wally was a conscientious objector who refused to serve in World War II. Initially, he was one of tens of thousands of Americans who spent time in a Civilian Public Service camp, where objectors had to perform civilian tasks in lieu of service. But after a year, he grew tired of the place and simply walked off one afternoon to make his way to Detroit. The government made sure to catch up with Wally. When he was arrested, Juanita got a call to go report the story. The two had been inseparable ever since.

Rose was no third wheel. She was a famous high jumper who only three years earlier had rejected an offer to join the United States track team in a match-up against the Soviet Union. She didn't want to be paraded around, to give the rest of the world the impression that Black American athletes were being treated equally. In 1959, she attended the Pan American Games in Chicago with thousands of athletes from two dozen countries. As the United States national anthem began to play over the speakers during the opening ceremony, similar worries crossed her mind. Rose made the decision not to stand.

The three waited outside the diner, hungry, and were joined by a white friend from Chicago named Kay Fields. The four entered and sat down peacefully. A waitress walked up and said, "We don't serve colored."

For a moment, they were frozen in shock. They had done sit-ins together many times before. They just hadn't planned this one. As a kid at age sixteen, Juanita had once been so humiliated sitting in the Jim Crow car of a train traveling from Cincinnati to Georgia that she got up to run around each train car testing out the seats. The porter, a Black man, had followed her, pleading with her to go back to her designated car, afraid that something would happen to the two of them. Sitting here at the Bar-H Chuck House on Route 40, it seemed like so little had changed.

The friends agreed they would wait in their seats together for twenty or thirty minutes, just to prove a point. Hardly five minutes had passed by the time two police officers arrived on the scene. "Show me your driver's license." Juanita refused. "I think I was really stalling because it hurt me so much to comply with this," she said. State troopers took the three Philadelphians to jail for trespassing. Kay Fields was allowed to stay, but she followed them out.

Juanita fought with the officers the entire way to jail. When they arrived, they placed twisters on her wrists—handcuffs with sharp points that would slice into her skin with every twist and pull. She hollered, demanding to go home. The police asked to fingerprint her. When she, Wally, and Rose refused, officers grabbed their hands and forced open their fingers.

Kay wasn't going to leave her friends behind. She arrived at Elkton Jail and turned herself in. Her hearing lasted only thirteen minutes. She was found guilty of trespassing and ordered to pay a fine, which she did before returning to Chicago.

Juanita, Wally, and Rose remained in jail in Elkton. They stopped eating, they refused to walk to the courtroom, and they would not respond to their charges. The courts grew desperate; demonstrators were showing up outside and the local news had started to talk about the three who had been arrested for simply trying to eat. For twelve days the friends, who had stopped at a restaurant only fifty miles from their home, continued to refuse to eat or cooperate. They told officials that they would "rather die" than respond to the court.

"We hope," fifty-two-year-old Wallace Nelson told reporters at the

Baltimore Afro-American, "that it will say something to the people of Maryland, that it will say that these laws [supporting discrimination] have got to go."

Weak from starvation and refusing to walk, the three were physically carried to jail for their hearing. In front of magistrate Leonard Lockhart, the defendants once again refused to enter a plea. The magistrate, angered by their refusal to respond to his questions, set a trial date for September 11, 1961. The state's attorney, J. Albert Roney Jr., realized he had another carceral option. To the court, the three resistors were intractable. The Elkton jail did not have the power to force them to eat—but a mental institution might.

Juanita, Wally, and Rose were taken from their cells and thrown into a police car with no notice, no explanation. One after another, they demanded to know where they were being taken. Finally, an officer replied. They were on their way to Crownsville Hospital.

Judge Edward D. E. Rollins of the Cecil County Circuit Court had ordered Sheriff Edgar Startt to commit the three to Crownsville. Startt told the *Baltimore Sun*, "Anybody that will not eat and won't stand up

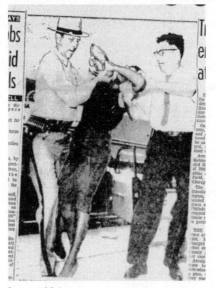

Juanita Nelson resists appearing in court.
Photo from the *Afro-American* newspaper.

in court and plead acts like a mental case to me—and also to the State's attorney."

All Juanita could think was, "Oh my Lord, they'll bury us there and nobody will ever know where we are," according to tapes held by the Memorial Hall Museum.

When they arrived at the hospital, Superintendent Charles Ward came out to greet them, rolling along wheelchairs to help bring them to their assigned rooms in the Medical Surgical Building. He wanted no part in this charade, but believed he had to show the state he was willing to do an evaluation. The very next day, he reported to the Cecil County Circuit Court that the Elkton Three were of sound mind and intelligence.

The portrayal of the case in the mainstream and Black press diverged significantly. The Elkton Three were depicted either as obstinate, childish individuals potentially suffering from insanity, or as citizens genuinely advocating for their civil rights. The *Baltimore Sun* and *Washington Post* did not debate segregation and restaurant discrimination and instead concentrated on the trio's refusal to cooperate with state officials. One *Baltimore Sun* article described the three friends as having been "carried by the sheriff's deputies" and as having "failed to cooperate." The article did not mention that their noncooperation was part of a civil rights protest, and seemed to portray the protesters as juvenile and stubborn in the face of neutral laws. Another *Washington Post* article described the protesters as unwilling "to walk two blocks from the jail to the courtroom." The piece glossed over most details of the case, but the emphasis on the "two blocks" distance to the courtroom left readers with the impression that the protesters were childish and their complaints were absurd.

The *Baltimore Afro-American* argued in a series of articles that the trio's arrest and mental hospital commitment were calculated attempts at silencing their civil rights, and discussed the three friends' determination to peacefully protest discrimination.

Black reporters took Maryland leaders to task. An opinion piece published on September 30, 1961, titled "One Way to Get in a Mental Hospital" challenged the state's attempts to label Black protesters as insane to discredit them. It read:

In most states they don't send sane people to mental hospitals, but here in the highly civilized state of Maryland, anything is liable to happen...In some sections of Maryland...white folks seem to think that when colored folks don't act like they (the white folks) think they should act, then the colored folks are crazy.

Superintendent Dr. Charles Ward's letter to the court, published in the *Afro-American*, provided a meticulous explanation of why the protesters had valid objections to their treatment. Dr. Ward concluded, "These people were appropriately dressed. They were well oriented as to time, place, and person. Their spirits appeared good...There was no evidence of delusional thinking or hallucinations of any type." Black reporters saw clearly that the Elkton Three were being labeled as "crazy" not because they displayed symptoms of any genuine illness but simply because they had defied the expectations of police officers and white business owners.

Meanwhile, that first night on the ward, the Elkton Three fought through their drowsiness and dehydration to talk long into the night. Crownsville staff, aware of the spreading scandal, told the three they could invite all the visitors that they wanted. They also promised not to force-feed them. Only one staff psychiatrist, a Holocaust survivor, seemed to be frustrated with them. "You're killing yourselves because you're not eating, and you should eat!" he allegedly shouted.

No evidence could be found that these friends were mentally ill, and within a few days, officers returned to the hospital to transport them back to jail. Juanita remembered Dr. Ward asking the group to please cooperate and to walk themselves out to the front of the hospital for the sake of the other patients there. They were grateful to him for his kindness and did as he asked. Back in the hands of police officers, they were found guilty of disorderly conduct and released after paying fines a few days later.

All the Elkton Three did was pull off Route 40 to buy a meal. Their resistance was nothing more than seeking rest and basic human treatment. But they had crossed both physical and invisible color lines, and the punishment for that in the South was not just public shame—it was a portrait of insanity. Crownsville had become a weapon against those who dared oppose the existing order.

Why We Go Crazy

At the very moment that the Elkton Three were incarcerated and court-committed to Crownsville, the truth in America's major metropolitan areas—once seemingly prosperous centers of manufacturing work and stable middle-class life—was beginning to unmask itself during the Civil Rights Movement. Millions of Black American families, just like my father's, had migrated to cities across the country in search of economic advancement, but open segregation and restrictive covenants in these majority-white communities forced them to settle into segregated and systematically underserved enclaves. These same restrictive, segregationist covenants meant that although Black people could find work in the Fordist industrial economy, they were given only the most hazardous and underpaid occupations available. It was these forces that brought my great-grandfather Clarence to an emotional and mental breaking point, and that led generations of Black organizers to lead protests, push for legislative reform, and publicly mourn the assassination of Black leaders. To put it simply: Black Americans refused to quiet their pain or to live as second-class citizens any longer.

The backlash was swift, and American urban spaces became criminalized to a sweeping extent. Behaviors that had once been associated with poverty and illness became part of a growing list of crimes that could land you in jail. The list included urinating in public, sleeping outside, begging for food, and consuming food on the train. A new preoccupation with crime not only expanded its definition but also reconfigured crime-fighting methods. In 1965, new federal commitments to fighting crime allowed local law enforcement to receive an influx of funds and equipment if they could show that crime was rising. In 1968, the Supreme Court decided *Terry v. Ohio*, a landmark ruling that found it was constitutional for police to stop and frisk a person they reasonably suspected to be armed and involved in a crime. The ruling made it easier for law enforcement officials to act on suspicion and "probable cause."

As many historians have previously argued, rising hostility toward Black protest and criminality fostered much of this new enthusiasm for expansive policing initiatives—and those initiatives were often narrowly aimed at America's Black citizens. Just as the neighbors of Maryland's Crownsville Hospital had feared Black patients' escape and riots to a degree that was disproportionate to their actual occurrence in the asylum system, so, too, did the white American electorate grossly overestimate the threat of Black crime. When there were riots, they very rarely came to white neighborhoods. Very few rioters attacked white people, and most of the casualties were caused by the police, not Black people protesting for social change. Meanwhile, the police were arresting peaceful protesters for bus boycotts, sit-ins, carpooling, or walking across the infamous Edmund Pettus Bridge in Selma.

Politicians like Governor George Wallace of Alabama, the man who authorized state troopers to beat and detain civil rights protesters on that very bridge in 1965, famously reached office by amplifying the racial anxieties of white voters. Wallace legendarily admitted that his political career took off after he focused on citizens' fears of Black people instead of on infrastructural improvements to the state: "You know, I tried to talk about good roads and good schools and all these things that have been part of my career, and nobody listened. And then I began talking about niggers, and they stomped the floor."

The Civil Rights Movement made criminality a disproportionately prevalent and racialized issue, setting in motion a pattern of events that stretched the definition of criminal behavior and strengthened every part of the carceral apparatus. Asylums included.

No form of medicine is immune to societal influence and manipulation. But the study and treatment of mental illness became especially vulnerable at that time. The field was essentially still in the Dark Ages— doctors were only just discovering medications and testing them out on patient populations that were warehoused, disorganized, long mistreated, and frequently misdiagnosed. Anxieties about race, resistance, and societal change crept into psychiatry and reshaped everything about the clinical context for all patients, not just African Americans. The Elkton Three were an example of this kind of infiltration, an early sign that some white leaders and doctors would, wittingly or unwittingly, misread Black anger as mental illness and use tools of psychiatry to punish, not to heal, the communities they were meant to serve.

Or, in stories like my family's, inequality and racial violence had the power to cause an unraveling and to sow the seeds of mental illness. And when those Black patients then sought help, they were, at times, met by psychiatric professionals who were not only unable to relate to their lived experiences—they saw their illness as evidence that white doctors had been right about Black patients all along.

In his book *The Protest Psychosis*, Jonathan Metzl documents a series of transformations from the 1940s through the 1970s, tracing how everything from patient diagnostic standards to pharmaceutical marketing underwent "rhetorical transformations" for schizophrenia and other debilitating mental illnesses, with a tendency to illustrate Black patients as uniquely hostile and belligerent. Prior to the Civil Rights Movement, the psychiatric Establishment viewed schizophrenia as a disease of disharmony—not violence—that primarily affected the white middle class or emotionally unbalanced housewives. Focusing on patient records from Michigan's Ionia State Hospital for the Criminally Insane, Metzl compared the descriptions of white and Black people with schizophrenia in the 1960s. He found that in 1965, the characteristic charts the doctors had made to describe white people with schizophrenia used language like: "limited ability to relate, friendly, cooperative, passive, unenergetic, manneristic, withdrawn, flat affect, childish thinking, inappropriate use of words, quiet, well adjusted, does not create any problems, low intelligence, slow speech, fears sexual contact, feels inadequate, paranoid, persecutory ideation: 'I think the police dept [*sic*] and judge are against me.'"

In 1966, Black patients' charts read: "dangerous, volatile, persecutory delusions, antisocial, disposed toward violence with minimal provocation, assaultive, drug dependent, paranoid, suspicious, hostile, very disturbed

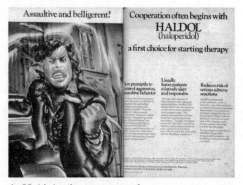

A Haldol advertisement features a menacing Black man who makes a fist as he hangs from a burning building in 1974. During the Civil Rights Movement, a growing number of Black men were diagnosed as schizophrenic. *Archives of General Psychiatry.*

individual, feels outside of society, aggressive impulses under tenuous control 'that could break down suddenly at anytime.'"

Metzl found that clinicians started to depict Black mental patients as threatening and uncontrollable, while white patients with the same illness were described sympathetically as "withdrawn," nonviolent, and compliant. Suddenly, the rates of schizophrenia among Black men skyrocketed, and the entire image of the disease changed. The title of Metzl's book came from a 1968 piece in *Archives of General Psychiatry*, in which two psychiatrists redefined schizophrenia as "a protest psychosis" that involved Black patients who had become hostile, aggressive, and developed "delusional anti-whiteness" after listening to leaders like Malcolm X or showing interest in the practice of Islam.

In one particularly heartbreaking section, Metzl lays out a series of correspondence between a Black family and the administration at Ionia Hospital. The family writes to the hospital to plead for their loved one, Otis, an army veteran, to be released or transferred to a hospital closer to their home. "My brother Otis was attacked by three persons in the street and managed to struggle and defend himself and fight back...Police officers were called or happened to the scene. As it was told to me, it appeared as if Otis was attacking the people...Miraculously he survived, totally unable to understand any part of this INSANE experience, he now begs for his life from the state mental institution," a family member wrote in their first letter, in February 1972, addressed to the Honorable Doctors at Ionia Hospital.

Over the course of nineteen months, letters were traded back and forth, and the family's anguish grew. At first, doctors politely denied Otis a release, even after criminal charges had been dropped against him for the fight. But by December 12, 1973, they wrote a letter to the patient's brother in definitive, impatient terms, uninterested in the family's description of Otis as someone who had actually been the victim of violence and unfairly profiled by the police. The doctors claimed that Otis was "unpredictable, threatening, and has required seclusion and close supervision. His thinking is confused and unrealistic, and he appears to be hallucinating. Although our diagnostic evaluation has not yet been completed, his condition is tentatively diagnosed as that of schizophrenia."

A few days later, on December 20, a private hospital progress note showed that a doctor at Ionia had described Otis as "uncooperative." He listed one volatile emotion after the other, providing little context or description of incidents or errors the patient had made. "He appears dangerous...speaks constantly of the Black Muslim group...sexually he is weak and inadequate...Prognosis is poor."

Research continues to find that psychiatrists are more likely to diagnose Black men with schizophrenia and that Black people are more likely to be prescribed antipsychotic medications—and at higher doses. In a 2018 meta-analysis of fifty-two different studies, researchers Charles Olbert, Arundati Nagendra, and Benjamin Buck found that Black Americans are 2.4 times more likely to be diagnosed with schizophrenia than white Americans. Back in 2014, a separate study found clear patterns in which Black Americans were diagnosed at a rate three to four times as high as white people, and Latino Americans were diagnosed at a rate more than three times higher than white Americans.

There's also the challenge of the persistent myths and stereotypes that shroud people who live with mental illness. There is often the assumption that people with diagnoses like schizophrenia are the most likely among us to commit acts of violence and become hardened criminals. The truth is, they are far, far more likely to be the victims than the perpetrators.

It doesn't help that psychiatry continues to be a field dominated by white doctors and nurses, many of them concentrated in communities with few ties to Black neighborhoods and culture. The number of Black doctors available remains out of step with the Black population in the U.S. and the number of patients who are seeking their help. The American Psychiatric Association's data shows that only 2 percent of the estimated 41,000 psychiatrists in the U.S. are Black, and just 4 percent of psychologists (who cannot prescribe medication, but often work with psychiatrists to do so) are Black.

We continue to live with the political and clinical consequences of our conflation of protest and madness. Juanita, Wally, and Rose may have been able to leave Crownsville and return to their normal lives in a matter of weeks, but only at an immense cost to themselves, their health, and their broader community in Maryland—who watched as their freedoms and aspirations were discredited at the highest levels in their state.

Almost two decades before the Elkton Three were court-committed to Crownsville for attempting to dine at a white-owned restaurant, an editorial published in the *Baltimore Afro-American* posed many of the same aching questions. In January 1947 the unnamed author of an article titled "Why We Go Crazy" offered his or her admittedly nonscientific analysis for why so many African Americans were being sent to asylums.

After noting that psychiatric experts had discussed the disproportionate rates of mental disease among Blacks, the author offered "a few contributing factors" for our consideration:

Colored persons always come up on the short end of jobs and pay...They ride the rear seats of many interstate buses, trains and boats because an outmoded Jim Crow law is still on the statute books. Some stores in Baltimore refuse to serve them at all, while others take their money, but employ them only as broom pushers. They get the worst housing and pay the most for it. Merely sitting down and thinking about these and countless other things just as bad in a nation that is trying to sell the world on the democratic way of life could drive a lot of people crazy, and it probably does.

CHAPTER 16

Sympathy for Me but Not Thee

A poem by a patient at Crownsville:

And from the ashes the phoenix will rise to smite out the death that come from the skies. Genocide in Korea, Vietnam and the rest trying to prove whose nation is best. The blood on the ground all liquid and the red screams of the dying, the stench of the dead.

THE ELKTON THREE MAY HAVE BEEN A PARTICULARLY BIZARRE AND public embarrassment for the state of Maryland, but that case provided an early and thorough example of patterns that were about to come into clear view throughout the 1960s and beyond. Civil rights and fundamental freedoms were at the center of the American consciousness. Decades of reporting had established the huge challenges facing mental hospitals and violations happening inside them. And now a pharmaceutical revolution was on the march. People were *supposed* to be feeling more sympathy and understanding toward patients with mental illness, and philosophers, filmmakers, and writers like Ken Kesey in *One Flew over the Cuckoo's Nest* were questioning the Establishment and seeking to empower patients. A change had come, and Crownsville—existing along the spectrum of asylum and jail and warehouse—was at the very center of the cultural negotiations that set the boundaries of how far, and to whom, that newfound sympathy would go.

In the mid-1950s so-called wonder drugs arrived from Europe. And within a few years of their introduction to the United States, they were everywhere in public and private practice. Thorazine, the brand name for the drug chlorpromazine, was first synthesized by the Rhone-Poulenc labs in France in 1950. In 1952, the first American clinical trials began. By 1956, more than three thousand patients in Maryland's system were being treated with the "new drugs," and more than four million Americans were using them, too. Not long after Thorazine, other antipsychotics and antidepressants were pumped out onto the market.

These psychiatric drugs fostered widespread hope for the rehabilitation of patients and encouraged communities to welcome loved ones back home. Their effects seemed, at first, nothing short of miraculous, and that's because they did more than just chemically lobotomize or stupefy previously aggressive patients. They allowed patients to keep their consciousness and intellect intact. No more screaming, no more wailing, fewer physical struggles on the wards. But doctors could lean on the medication to engage the patient in their own therapy. Before antipsychotics, treatment—which ranged from moral and emotional engagement with patients to somatic procedures like electroshock or lobotomy—was largely perceived to fail and often required intense physical involvement from staff in institutions. Now, physicians and families could report quieter hospital wards and lasting improvements to patient convalescence, leading them to gain confidence that the mentally ill could return home without hardship to themselves or their families. Pretty quickly, the social emphasis was no longer on how best to eradicate mental illness for the benefit of society, but rather on how society may be better able to serve and accommodate its mentally ill.

That increasingly optimistic and sympathetic climate of the mid-twentieth century set the stage for deinstitutionalization, or the mass patient exodus from asylums. In 1963, the push for community-centered care came to the forefront as United States president John F. Kennedy announced the Community Mental Health Act.

For him, matters of mental health and disability were personal. His parents had kept the story and whereabouts of his intellectually disabled older sister, Rosemary, hidden from the public for years. After years of learning struggles, she became incapacitated after their father sent her for a botched lobotomy in 1941. The procedure left her with the mental capacity of a two-year-old, and she was institutionalized for decades. The Kennedys brushed off any questions about her absence during JFK's political campaigns by claiming that she was a recluse. But just two years after he became president, in a special message to Congress in February 1963, JFK outlined a new mode of mental healthcare, one that would give patients like his sister a fighting chance to be treated with dignity and to stay close to home.

"Central to a new mental health program is comprehensive community care," Kennedy said in a special address to Congress. "Merely pouring federal funds into a continuation of the outmoded type of institutional care which now prevails would make little difference." In place of the old asylum model, he announced, there would soon be more flexible, locally accessible healthcare services. Essentially, the government would act as a cash reserve or early investor, with the expectation that states would ultimately build, sustain, and lead these programs. "We need a new type of health facility, one which will return mental healthcare to the mainstream of American medicine, and at the same time upgrade mental health services," the president declared.

Only a few years later under President Lyndon B. Johnson, the introduction of the federal Medicaid program doubled down on its displacement of the asylum. Medicaid contained explicit incentives to keep patients out of state institutions by denying medical coverage to those who remained inside them. American psychiatric opinion embraced the logic of deinstitutionalization, once described by social workers Martin Wolins and Yochanan Wozner as the belief that "people are made into healthy humans by their interaction with a competent social environment" and not in institutions. That ethos was made clear in advertisements. Thorazine ran an advertisement carrying the tag line "Thorazine helps to keep more patients out of mental hospitals" and made explicit the clinical goal of using medication to reintegrate patients with their communities. It included a photograph of several men who each appeared to be out on their regular commute to work or running errands in a plaza.

Drug advertisements would argue that a community-based environment is a far better alternative to the old model of institutional dependence, and that drugs like Thorazine opened previously closed lines of communication between patients, clinics, and communities.

But as the Elkton Three's case shows, the state could still make inappropriate use of its various carceral apparatuses to detain the civil rights demonstrators in a way that was not consistent with a newfound focus on community or with the nationwide push to stop using the asylum as a receptacle. It was more consistent with law and order and the status quo. There was a strange tension, or contradiction: at the same time that society became less and less invested in large-scale institutional mental healthcare, many people remained enveloped by their fears of Black criminals and protesters, and so other, less high-profile patients at Crownsville got caught somewhere in between.

One summer afternoon, an alarm rang out in the Hugh Young Building. Staff needed to mobilize. A patient was up on the roof.

The supervisor and nurse on the scene, Delores Hawkins, was used to this kind of thing. The patients assigned to her tended to be women who had been labeled as violent, unreachable, and chaotic. Many of them had been sexually and physically abused by family members or partners, and had found their way to Crownsville through one of two systems: the foster care system or the criminal legal system. Delores was skinny and all of five feet, three inches. She didn't look like the kind of person who could carry an adult patient down off the roof. But she had a cheeky smile and big, deep-set brown eyes, and she maintained a kind of eye contact that made it easy for her to connect and to disarm people. She was known to listen, not fight—the kind of nurse who built deep relationships with her patients.

She took a deep breath. She had no business going up on a roof. She hated heights. Still, Delores made her way up three flights of stairs to a low-pitched sloping hipped roof. She looked out, and there was a patient named Ramona, cackling.

Ramona had been in Crownsville for as long as anyone could remember. Unlike Delores, it seemed like she was ten feet tall. Ramona controlled her own schedule at the hospital and ate her meals when she wanted to. She received a special private room after administrators identified her as someone with the potential to start a riot, someone who would not be a calming influence on the women's dormitory. Staff had been told that she was psychotic, but they couldn't find any evidence for that. In fact, she seemed to know more about the place than they did. When male attendants came by her floor, she'd wink and lie down on the floor. She knew who was hooking up with whom, and she would tattle to the supervisors when one of their colleagues took a nap on their shift. She seemed to always know when there was tension brewing between patients and staff. She would lean her head out the window of HY Building and yell at other patients and employees. "Hey, you tell them people up there in Cottage 15 that my friend better not get hurt." Delores had immense respect for Ramona. She tried to hide that she feared her.

Delores took one step out onto the roof. Of course, Ramona had chosen a perch on the oldest part of the Hugh Young Building's roof—the section first constructed in 1925. All Delores's deeply religious self could do was pray. And curse a little bit. She couldn't believe they had put her out there.

"Why don't you come inside? Come on, now. Please. For God's sake. Let's head down." Delores began visibly shaking, clinging to the edge of a roof that everyone knew could use some repairs. She had never seen the building from this angle. It was an imposing central structure, visible to people from the street, fifteen bays wide and seven bays deep. Boy, it was a long way down.

Colleagues had gathered on the top floor and out on the grass to help—or to watch. Ramona was enjoying every minute of it. From up there, you could look out at all of Crownsville's campus. Ramona could take in all of this little city within a town that had become her home. Ramona had never really been free. Before Crownsville, she had been incarcerated at a nearby prison. Before that, all the staff knew was that Ramona had been mixed up with some very abusive men. As Delores came to understand, she was searching for these small moments—when she could bend a rule, breathe some air on her own terms for once.

After what felt like an eternity, Ramona called out to her audience. "All right. Let me take this fool inside before she kills herself." Ramona walked across the sloping roof, lifted Delores up off the ground, and carried her nurse back to safety inside.

Years later, when I sat with Delores, Gertrude Belt, and their friends for lunch, I got the sense that they missed Ramona, that they worried about where she was now. They looked back on their time with her fondly, almost as though she was a stubborn, rambunctious friend they had lost touch with. But as the years passed, they explained, Ramona's battles with administrators became more and more pronounced. The administration didn't find incidents like the one on the roof to be comical, or interpret them as a call for a little more freedom or space. The bedroom that Ramona had all to herself eventually became a personal prison, as word came down from administrators that Ramona was not to be allowed to do anything without a minimum of four employees present to escort her.

Gertrude was one of the people assigned to regularly walk her to and from the shower. She still has vivid memories of coming up to Ramona, who would be standing in her room in seclusion, and trying to exchange a supportive smile. Gertrude believed the administration wanted to make an example out of patients like her.

"She knew too much," Gertrude told me as Delores sat next to her and looked down. "They could not do to her what they had done to the others."

When Crownsville eventually closed down decades later, Ramona was reassigned to a different correctional facility. The women who had worked with her at Crownsville never talked to her again. At the table, there was an open question of why Ramona, as well as other patients they had spent years working with, had never made it out. She was not one of the patients who were unable to bathe or dress themselves, unable to stick to a medication regimen. Sure, she broke rules and didn't like to eat when told to. But, to them, that hardly seemed like a sign someone was so sick or hopelessly dangerous that they couldn't ever make their way home again. Even if she had no home or family, that didn't mean she could not find one. It seemed like there was one story in the press and another story on the private wards. There were the patients in the Thorazine ads, mostly white, who were indeed going to find their way back to their community. But many of the patients at Crownsville might never be judged well enough to get released.

Delores's time at Crownsville can be characterized as one of extremes and contradictions. She was witness to some of the most carceral impulses of the time, but she was also tasked, on paper, with making community mental health a priority. Much of her job focused on adolescents and family relationships, guided by a philosophy popular in the sixties and seventies that believed patients were a symptom of larger failings in the family structure. Healing them, therefore, required her to make sure that the connection between the family and the patient was not broken. She would set up regular meetings with parents and act like a negotiator, trying to find windows when it would be okay for the child to come home and visit. This was the entire point of the new focus on community mental health treatment.

Community healthcare, of course, rests on the assumption that there is a community that will welcome someone home. But sometimes the reality that Delores saw was bleak. The most vulnerable people were those abandoned at Crownsville precisely because they had no one in their corner. Many came from poorer neighborhoods where they had no access to a good clinic or physician with whom Crownsville could coordinate care. Sometimes there was no family to call, or the family was the patient's abuser. This was why the hospital had found itself at the center of the civil rights debate. The same forces of racism, poverty and unemployment, and social alienation that activists like the Elkton Three sought to dismantle were shaping and complicating the work of Crownsville staff every day.

One of the teenage patients Delores worked with had been in and out of different foster homes because she was always fighting. Every time the young girl was placed somewhere new, she wound up punching someone and getting kicked out. Eventually, she wound up at Crownsville.

Delores and the patient were walking the grounds one day when the teen punched her straight in the face with no warning. Delores stumbled, confused. Then she drew her own fists up to her chin in a boxing stance, ready to swing back if she had to. "Have you lost your mind?" she shouted.

"But I love you," the girl replied.

Now Delores was deeply confused. She sat the girl down and asked her why on earth she would punch someone that she loves. The girl told her about her parents and foster parents. She described how every last one of them beat her at home but then would tell her that they loved her or that it was all going to be okay. She didn't think getting punched was a big deal. She thought physical violence was an appropriate, funny way of expressing love.

Delores didn't have the option of meeting with this patient's family, and wouldn't have pushed for her to be returned to them even if that had been on the table. She was well aware of what would happen to a young Black girl who continued on the current path. So Delores adjusted her treatment plan and started intense behavior modification work, focused on positive reinforcement to restore her self-esteem. Today, that young girl is a wife and mother of three children. She and Delores would catch up on the phone every year or so. While their relationship was a reflection of the healing power of listening and therapy, it was also a reminder to Delores of how much her job depended on her to become a stand-in for a concept of community and resources that often just didn't exist. That child could have become Ramona —locked up in a seclusion cell, labeled as deviant or hopeless by administration, and cycled from one institution to the next, with no chance of benefiting from the broader social trends that were meant to transform their lives.

While there are many accounts of patients successfully coming home and families feeling whole again, that was not the case for some of the

Black children and adults who entered Crownsville. Staff at Crownsville desperately wanted their patients to recover and enjoy the full rights and benefits of a society that claimed it was ready to reintegrate them back home. But they also knew that society tended to break its promises to people who looked like them. In 1960, the hospital's superintendent, Charles Ward, wrote in one report that "the day of the large expanding State Hospital seems to be over and it is my belief that we can now work towards our own eventual dissolution." But that shift—even in the best scenario—was going to take place over the long term. He did not buy the broader narrative that new medication and funding were the silver bullet to every patient's problems. "The return of the patients to the community such as has been accomplished does not necessarily mean that those patients are improved or that their individual illnesses have been altered," he warned.

So much of the duality in Crownsville is evident throughout the 1960s. Records and newspapers from the 1960s show that state leaders still welcomed the use of the asylum, when convenient, as a repository for the criminalized populations it struggled to detain elsewhere. For Crownsville, it always seemed to be one step forward, one step back. The hospital, for example, established its first outpatient clinic in Baltimore in 1961 with the hope of preventing relapse in some of its discharged patients. But in that same year, the State Department of Corrections attempted, though ultimately failed, to acquire 159 acres of land belonging to Crownsville "for use as a prison camp," according to *Baltimore Sun* reporter Stuart S. Smith. The prison camp in question had been previously located on Department of Forests and Parks land, but the department reportedly wanted the camp to relocate so that a park could be further developed for recreational purposes. Though Crownsville patients were not regularly using the proposed acres, the administration warned that it would be a "potential hazard" to add the prison camp and its traffic to the hospital's grounds. Anne Arundel commissioner Louis Boehm questioned why the state chose Crownsville instead of Jessup, where there was lots of available land and where a women's correctional institution had been established. He asked, "Why don't they move it right up to Jessup?"

Throughout the sixties, the line between patient and inmate, criminal or insane, continued to get blurred. At one point in 1969, there was intense public debate over the consideration of a bill that would allow citizens to ask police officers to forcibly commit another person to an asylum. A *Baltimore Sun* article from January 29, 1969, titled "Bill to Commit Deranged Filed" explained that a proposed piece of legislation "would allow any person to file a petition with a 'state or local peace officer,' asking that another person be committed to a mental institution. With the corroboration of two physicians, the person complained of can be committed for up to fourteen days." Two of the four people included in the commitment process—the layperson/accuser and peace officer—had no medical or mental health credentials at all. Some worried that the bill aimed to empower fearful and anxious locals rather than sincerely serve those potentially in need of institutional care.

That same year, Crownsville superintendent Dr. George Phillips spoke to the Baltimore *Evening Sun* in an effort to humanize his patients and the work of his staff. The reporter opened the piece with a zinger: "Unlike the dark side of the moon which few people see, the dark side of a mental hospital stands out." Dr. Phillips urged the reporter and readers to not think of "mental patients as people who have to be locked up." He told them their doors were open, that community members should come visit and see their operations—like the evening group therapy they provided to both patients and their parents.

The blurred lines between the asylum and the prison came into view that year, when a series of articles and op-eds argued over the court commitment of a thirty-nine-year-old woman forced to stay at Crownsville for sixty-four days, sparking candid conversations about the involvement of law enforcement in mental health proceedings. The case, reported in the *Baltimore Sun*, involved a woman who was sent to Crownsville after her son accused her of making a "nuisance telephone call to him." Forty-one days passed inside Crownsville before she was seen by a psychiatrist, and when she was finally released, she returned home to find her food business was ruined. As one delegate remarked at the time: landing in Crownsville was not unlike jail, "as they are actually losing their liberties."

The treatment of that woman was not a unique or isolated incident. In fact, the director of forensic psychiatry at Crownsville, Dr. Osker T. Koryak, went on the record saying that many defendants had been confined at Crownsville for periods of sixty days or longer as a result of court orders and that 90 percent had been returned to the courts with certification that they were competent. In other words, officials used the asylum as a waiting room for the accused, with an astounding error rate and with the added result that by virtue of their (sometimes dubious) status as insane persons, the person held would lose the right to live and work privately until their arraignment. One excerpt from the 1969 *Baltimore Sun* piece "Slipshod Justice for Mental Cases" by A. W. Geiselman Jr. speaks for itself:

By far the most urgent issue is what Thomas J. Curley, chief judge of the Anne Arundel County People's Court, describes as "the emergency detention and commitment of individuals believed to be dangerous by reason of mental health." Judge Curley... has been pushing for "emergency" legislation for at least three years with no success. He concedes that his court has sent scores of persons charged with minor crimes to Crownsville State Hospital since July 1, 1966, using a 1968 law that doesn't apply to many of these defendants. The Legislature won't give him the law he needs to get these "dangerous" people off the street; therefore he has used such law as is available, questionable though this might be... Judge Curley points out that for years the accepted method of getting a person committed to a mental hospital when he didn't want to be committed was for a relative or friend to file a minor criminal charge against him, such as disorderly conduct, disturbing the peace, or assault. Everyone knew that these were contrived charges, in many cases completely fictitious, but the charges resulted in the recalcitrant subject being snapped up by police, taken to a judge and then off to the mental hospital.

Judge Curley's hope was that lawmakers would pass a bill that gave courts the right to order law enforcement to take someone into custody who was living with mental illness and possibly dangerous. It would ideally be a civil and not a criminal matter. He acknowledged that he had court-committed people to Crownsville who may not have committed any crimes and who had not been processed by standard psychiatric procedures. The reader is left wondering if and how the woman accused of making a nuisance telephone call to her son fits into the category of "dangerous" people. Curley was the judge who had committed her.

Paul Lurz and about a dozen other employees told me this was an open secret. Paul explained to me that not only was it common for judges and hospital psychiatrists to "never [seem] to be in a rush" to evaluate those committed but that it was also common for the Baltimore police to pick up the mentally ill and homeless and leave them in the city jail. Then, Paul explained, they would be transferred to Crownsville, and his team would receive medical certificates for the transfer that were always signed by the same two physicians using the identical wording. "The rumor was that they simply walked past the jail cells, looked in, then filled out the committing certificates" that immediately transferred people from the jail to the hospital.

At a time when the hospital was supposed to be focused on discharging patients and prioritizing bonds with families and communities, Crownsville was still an appendage to Maryland law enforcement, mediated by officers and judges who actively collaborated in a process that seemed to care little for distinctions like those between "mental illness" and "criminality." It was an imperfect appendage, though. While the label of mental illness expedited the state's confinement of many individuals, the work of employees like Delores often disrupted, slowed, or reversed it, protecting some patients from the worst outcomes.

Other social forces were about to reshape the hospital as well. In addition to revolutions in medical and institutional culture and the national fight for civil rights, the country was engaged in a war that would have no winners. And Black men from rural Georgia to East Baltimore were signing up to fight it.

War Comes Home

They would ride by patrol boat, hose in hand, or they would fly low, a hundred or so feet above the ground, in helicopters or small planes. Behind them, stretching for miles, was a white mist. It would hang in the air, like lines of chalk all across the greenery. Within a few weeks, that mist would turn much of what it touched to dust. The jungle would bow, green would turn to brown, and American soldiers would be able to make their way through. So effective, even in the rain it wouldn't be washed away. This war was entirely in jungle terrain. America's enemy—the Vietcong—knew it all intimately. The density of the foliage provided endless possibilities for guerilla warfare. American troops were in a constant, heightened state of panic in Vietnam, knowing their enemy could approach without being seen. To beat the North Vietnamese, they had to beat the jungle.

On November 30, 1961, President Kennedy approved the use of chemicals in Vietnam. Soon, fifty-five-gallon drums arrived on air bases, clearly marked with an identifying orange stripe.

The soldiers were assured this white mist wouldn't harm *them*. Barely clothed out in the mind-boggling heat, they would spray the mixture straight from their trucks, planes, or boats, right onto the riverbank or a rice field. It was called Agent Orange, and it was a fifty-fifty mix of two herbicides: 2,4,5-trichlorophenoxyacetic acid and 2,4-dichlorophenoxyacetic acid. Together, they acted as a chemical defoliant and weapon of war, depriving the enemy of both their cover and their food.

For a young Black man from Maryland, all of this might as well have been happening on another planet. Hell, another solar system. He was traveling through a land and climate that looked nothing like home, fighting shoulder to shoulder with white men—the kind who would've paid him no mind back in Baltimore. This was the first racially integrated war. On the surface, they all shared the same mission. Everything about that was surreal.

But Earth found ways to creep in around soldiers like him. After a few drinks, the N-word would start slipping out. White boys would scrawl horrifying graffiti in the barracks about killing their Black brothers-in-arms. Some hung the Confederate flag in the barracks and made their membership in the Ku Klux Klan plain. The racial tensions that had boiled over on American soil had traveled here to the tall elephant grass. They were moving through a foreign nation, carrying with them the responsibility to defend freedom and democracy. But would they even recognize it if they found it? How were they to defend something that they had never been able to experience for themselves?

As activists like the Elkton Three launched actions at home, Black soldiers found their ways to build power and call out hypocrisy, too. They would don Black amulets, beads, and accessories to represent their Black pride, and during downtime they would retreat into their own world, drinking together and listening to soul music.

At the start of 1965 there were under twenty-five thousand U.S. servicemen in Vietnam. By the end of 1968, there were half a million. The United States had dropped qualification standards for the draft, pulling in poor Blacks and poor whites who would have otherwise escaped it. Tensions only increased. African Americans were placed in ground combat battalions in higher percentages than whites, and while African Americans made up just over 10 percent of the general population in 1965, they suffered 24 percent of the U.S. Army's fatal casualties. Among Black soldiers a paranoid theory emerged: perhaps they were putting us on the front lines for genocidal purposes.

On February 25, 1967, Martin Luther King Jr. stood at a podium in Los Angeles and asked the nation to make a full accounting of the atrocities committed at home and abroad. "We see the rice fields of a small Asian country being trampled at will and burned at whim; we see grief-stricken mothers with crying babies clutched in their arms as they watch their little huts burst forth into flames; we see the fields and valleys of battle being painted with humankind's blood; we see the broken bodies left prostrate in countless fields; we see young men being sent home half-men—physically handicapped and mentally deranged."

That October in 1967, a number of Crownsville employees, including Paul Lurz, drove to Washington, D.C., and joined a hundred thousand people in a march on the Pentagon in protest of the war.

On the Crownsville campus, Dr. Errol Phillip, the Trinidadian psychiatrist, received the dreaded summons: he had been drafted to go to Vietnam. He was one of many doctors called to join the armed forces. But Errol was a permanent resident, not yet an American citizen, and he had three kids and dozens of patients to take care of.

He was writing notes at the nursing station one afternoon when one of his patients, Mr. Hall, walked in and asked him for a cigarette. Regrettably, Errol didn't have any to offer. He apologized and turned back to his papers as the patient walked away. He didn't think much of it—he'd been treating the man and his identical twin without incident. It was common for psychiatric patients to self-medicate by smoking, and doctors frankly didn't mind because the nicotine seemed to regulate their moods and alleviate some anxiety. It was so common that Maryland officials made a routine of swinging by Crownsville and dropping off packs of cigarettes that the state had confiscated from people who tried to ship them illegally across state lines. Errol didn't realize how badly his patient needed a smoke.

Moments later, Mr. Hall burst back into the room wielding an office chair. In a split second, Errol lifted his right hand to protect himself and one of the nurses. The chair came crashing down. With the help of staff, Errol got into a hospital car and was taken to the University of Maryland. There, he discovered that Mr. Hall had broken the trapezium bone in his wrist and another in his thumb.

When Errol eventually went downtown to fulfill his draft obligations, it was his injured wrist, combined with his age, that spared him from deployment. Reflecting on this memory during a conversation we had in April 2022, Errol sat there with a smile. "It was this!" his wife, Joyce, said as she pointed to her hand. "In a way, the patient almost saved him from going to Vietnam."

In April 1968, Martin Luther King Jr. would be assassinated in Memphis. Riots would break out in cities across America, and Baltimore was no exception. Faye Belt, who was just a teenager at the time, remembers walking through a cornfield that connected Crownsville's campus to her family's backyard, and hearing her sister, Frederica, shout from a window, "They shot Martin Luther King!" Her mom, Gertrude, could only describe the next day at work as sad and horrible.

In Vietnam, white superiors would break the news to their Black subordinates, but not before seizing their weapons to ensure none of the rage was turned back on them. Black soldiers were in shock. It seemed like the air had been sucked out of the jungle. They would mourn together, exhausted and reeling over the loss of a hero many of them had believed was capable of liberating them. They listened as white soldiers partied and joked in the distance. On some bases white boys paraded around, joking about the murder.

The physical and mental derangement that King had called out was obvious. Americans were growing angrier at the human cost of this war. But the chemical warfare—the eleven million gallons of mist that hung in the jungle, that burrowed into the soil and sunk under your skin— nobody had accounted for that yet.

The young Black man came home from the war to Baltimore, where his wife and brother lived. For all of the upheaval, so much at home had fundamentally remained the same. It was he who had changed. Once an energetic man who would spend time with his buddies at the boxing gym and had plans to build a family—now his personality was irritable and dark. He couldn't sleep. He couldn't find good paying work or hold down a job. His relationship with his wife was disintegrating.

Looking back, his brother suspected he had developed post-traumatic stress disorder. But he wasn't getting treatment and wasn't making progress adjusting to civilian life. As sociologist James M. Fendrich put it: Black Vietnam veterans came back to America and had to face "the transition from 'democracy in the foxhole' to discrimination in the ghetto at home." Their anger and alienation from American society was simmering, not dissipating. The military, as it turned out, was ahead of most large American institutions in its pace and willingness to integrate.

But for the men exposed to this toxin, there was also an underlying change in their health. Sometimes their memory was shot—their thinking often completely illogical. Their nerves and impulses could be jumpy and unpredictable. It could feel like their limbs were numb, or worse, on fire. The man from Maryland continued to dress in combat clothes and heavy black boots, as though any minute now he was going to be shipped back to the jungle. Everyone had read the stories about the terrible mist he had helped spray all across Vietnam. Hundreds of thousands of Vietnamese people died from Agent Orange exposure. An immeasurable number of families were harmed, and many of their children were born with congenital disabilities. It seemed the toxin not only altered the person exposed to it, it changed their DNA and their family's future. Chemicals powerful enough to destroy an ecosystem likely had the power to fundamentally reconfigure this soldier. At his brother's urging, the man walked into the Veterans Affairs office and filed a disability claim. Only to find it was denied.

When the family eventually got the news that he had exploded at his wife and murdered her, they knew that the man they loved had been completely consumed by the toxin.

One afternoon in the winter of 1999, Faye Belt walked across Crownsville's lawn to the far corner of the campus for her regular three p.m. shift in the two-floor brick cottages that had become home to some of the most challenging long-term patients. She left her only son, Jahmeal "Musa," whom she had nicknamed after the king of the ancient empire of Mali, at her mother's house that day. She was often anxious, finding it difficult to secure trustworthy childcare. She and her son's father weren't on the best of terms, and Faye was double-dipping, taking shifts at both Spring Grove Hospital and Crownsville.

She entered the front door of Cottage 12 into a ward organized like a cross. To the left was her supervisor's door, to the right the nursing station. She made her rounds, greeting patients and catching up on their charts. She noticed that several of them hadn't yet received their medications. She was pissed. And she made the other nurses aware of it.

As Faye walked around, something didn't feel right. Every time she turned her head, it felt like there were eyes on her. Like a patient was watching. A friend and fellow nurse came up to her in the hallway and asked to see a photo of Musa, who had just started in the third grade. Before Faye could pull her son's photo out of her pocket, she saw a shadow flicker in her peripheral vision.

Terrified, Faye turned. The shadow was hurtling straight toward her. The only image she can clearly recall is his deep-set eyes. They were brown and beautiful, but furious. Within seconds, a man was on top of her and had knocked her out cold with a massive fist.

Faye does not know if she screamed. She doesn't know how long she was unconscious underneath this man or how long it took for her training to kick in. When she came to on the floor, she saw her friend frozen above her. "Call the fucking code. Call it right now."

They called a silent code—ringing the nursing stations directly, alerting colleagues that Faye was in danger without the patients knowing.

A flurry of physicians and colleagues flooded the room. A doctor urgently advised everyone to subdue the patient and administer a series of medications. Faye, bruised and delirious, stumbled through the motions, forced into helping secure her own crime scene. There was no time to think or breathe. The doctor enlisted two nearby nurses and aides to help restrain the man. As they scrambled to hold down his arms and legs, the patient seemed to take the form of a shadow again, never taking his eyes off his target, writhing and contorting his body. He kicked Faye. She heard a loud pop and collapsed on the floor again. With a single kick, he had snapped her ACL and inner and outer meniscus bands.

Faye took more than a year of leave from work. I spoke to friends of hers, who donated their own vacation days to her so she could heal. She remembers coming home from the hospital in panic mode. She was in complete denial. The surgeon tried to rush her to surgery, but she refused for two weeks. She stumbled around her home with a cumbersome brace that locked everything from her ankle up to her hip, convinced she couldn't leave her son.

For days it felt like the snow just wouldn't stop. Musa, her little guy, was doing what he could to make her meals, struggling to wash the dishes. Her neighbors would come by to light fires for her. The house was a complete mess.

When she came back to Cottage 12 over a year later, the man was still there. Faye was terrified. She stayed as far away from him as she could and focused on tending to the other patients. She walked over to the TV and turned on some cartoons, hoping they would distract everyone and hide the fact that she was struggling to go through the motions. I was not able to locate a record of her assault, and the superintendent at the time, Ron Hendler, says leadership would have been required to file a police report and immediately transfer the patient out of the hospital. Several employees told me that while that was a rule at the time, it was rarely followed. Hendler told me, "If Faye said it happened, it happened."

One day the cottage doorbell rang. A man in a military uniform was waiting at the door. When he laid eyes on Faye, he let out a gasp. "Oh my God. You look just like her." It was the brother of the veteran from Baltimore. He asked Faye if they could talk.

Faye looked just like the patient's dead wife. According to the brother, he had seen Faye arrive that day in Cottage 12 and was convinced that she was a reincarnation of his wife, a reminder of the worst thing he had ever done. His brother talked with her about how the man left Maryland for Vietnam and came home an alien in his own land. How he had been given the runaround, denied healthcare. How he had been tasked with spraying Agent Orange across a country that had never harmed him, never denied him a job or assassinated his leaders. He explained how, worst of all, his brother didn't realize that in spraying a foreign people's land to death, he had killed himself. War had taken a physical, mental, and biochemical toll. The visitor wanted to apologize for his brother. He was amazed that Faye wasn't angry. All she did was cry uncontrollably.

Today, Faye harbors no anger toward the patient, though she doesn't make light of the harm he caused not only to her but also to his wife and community. He was eventually transferred from Crownsville to a maximum-security forensic psychiatry hospital and passed away from complications from Agent Orange exposure. In her view, he was a victim as much as she was. She had met Black men like him before, men whose country had sold their health and well-being for a false performance of democracy. Some of them were in her own family. She told me, "The military dropped the ball on their soldiers. They were not the same people. Some tried to be happy. But you eventually saw the mental illness."

I pushed her, asking why she wasn't angry with the patient at all. Even just a bit. He almost killed her after all. She shot back, "Why should I be?"

PART FIVE

Where Have All the Patients Gone?

1970–2004

1970: 1,620 Patients
2004: 200 Patients

CHAPTER 17

In the Balance

JUST BEFORE TWO P.M. ON A GRAY AND COLD FRIDAY AT THE END OF February 1972, Dr. George McKenzie Phillips, the first Black superintendent of a Maryland state hospital, sat in his office waiting for a handful of esteemed visitors to arrive on campus. Dr. Phillips was dynamic and confident, but strict. His facial expressions were known to reveal what he was thinking before he spoke. Every colleague of his describes observing the long hours he spent preoccupied about Crownsville's future. His daughter Lisa, who grew up on the campus, remembers believing her father was so distinguished that she struggled to make eye contact with him. In the evenings after work, his seven children would listen at the dinner table as he described the political realities he faced at the hospital and the "obstructionist" people who had made it challenging for him to get funding. He tried to live out his values in every area of his life, and he chose to enroll his children in the local public school instead of the private school used by the other doctors' families. "This concept was how he carried out his vision with mental health," his daughter Diane explained. "People with mental health deserve the same level of care and dignity like any other person in need of healthcare." He did not believe in private education, or in a mental healthcare system that was becoming increasingly out of reach.

The group visiting that afternoon had received complaints about the hospital's practices and wanted to see what was going on. Dr. Phillips, after years of being pulled in every direction as superintendent, a regional director for mental health, and a doctor in private practice, was more than happy to let this group experience Crownsville's honest condition for themselves. He wanted them to see just how difficult these last few years had been for his team, and to possibly help him fight for a solution. Their visit also offered him the chance to give them a piece of his mind.

Seven members of the governor's Humane Practices Commission entered—including its chairperson, John Kent, who was a delegate from Baltimore City; Dr. Paul Lemkau, the renowned chair of Johns Hopkins Department of Mental Hygiene; and other state lawmakers and disability advocates. There was not a single person of color. They filed behind Dr. Phillips as he walked them across the grounds and talked them through some basic facts.

Crownsville's population was now down to 1,033 patients, though there were beds for 1,172. Of the 1,033, 220 were geriatric, 80 of them considered "mentally retarded." He brought them first to the Winterode Building, where the hospital had been operating a school that was dealing with constant turnover, with a combination of day students from the community and patients at the hospital. The principal, an educator named Allen Brewington, took advantage of the opportunity and audience before him. He stood to speak to the delegation and told them that despite promises to the contrary, he was still receiving no state aid for his fledgling program. He had received some funds from the federal government, but there seemed to be some anxiety that those dollars would soon be on the chopping block, too.

Chairman Kent then pressed Dr. Phillips to take them to the Meyer Building—the commission had received a tip complaining about the use of seclusion rooms there, and he wanted to see them for himself. Dr. Phillips made no attempt to hide what was happening.

The members of the commission peered through tiny windows into three seclusion rooms. They saw three patients lying on bare mattresses on the floor. A patient called out to the commissioners, asking if they happened to have a blanket. No beds. No books. No furniture. The commission secretary scribbled down in her notebook: "No doors on toilets although there were toilet seats in this building."

Next they visited the "mentally retarded" patients housed in the basement of New Building. One of the commission members argued with the care team there, worried about the message being sent to the patients, who were striving to become more independent during the day, only to be returned to a locked ward each night. Dr. Phillips promised to look into moving them to a more open ward.

From there, they traveled to the Geriatrics building, where elderly patients were waiting in a basement dining room for food to arrive. The commission's secretary jotted down another note for the record: "The contrast between these patients at dinner and the [mostly white] geriatric patients at Eastern Shore State Hospital at dinner in the Choptank Room was appalling." The commissioners asked to talk with Dr. Phillips in his conference room. He obliged.

They argued about everything. From how there were forty-three job vacancies and no money for overtime, to a lack of funding for innovative programs, to whether Dr. Phillips had taken on too much responsibility. Dr. Phillips told them he was worried about patients who were leaving the hospital and receiving no follow-up care. He told them something Black staff had long discussed but never got to say to white state leaders' faces. He believed he knew why the legislature had never been truly committed to his hospital. The secretary wrote down in a report the commission filed as confidential: "He believes that this is because of Crownsville's history as originally the state facility for the Negro."

Things Fall Apart

Dr. Phillips was likely coming to terms with a new and somewhat shameful reality. The dream of community mental healthcare—that optimism that so defined the late fifties and early sixties—was crashing and burning. Patients were leaving hospitals and finding there were no clinics to visit. State lawmakers who had acted incensed when there were scandals at their local asylums and had celebrated the shrinking of state institutions were no longer raising their hands to fight for new projects. The rug was getting pulled out from under the system. It took a toll on Dr. Phillips, who would come back to the superintendent's house exhausted at night and make a beeline for his study. His daughter Diane would bring him his dinner. "The next day, bright and early, he was ready to face the next day's challenges," she told me. "I honestly believe that those who didn't agree with seeing mental health in a new way looked for ways to defeat his efforts regardless of their race."

By the mid to late 1960s there was mounting evidence that the state-federal partnership spurred by President Kennedy's 1963 Community Mental Health Act wasn't working as planned. Across the country, states were having difficulty meeting basic requirements mandated by federal law, and were having trouble finding state and local funds for construction and staffing to match a desired contribution from the federal government. As historian Jonathan Engel argued in a sprawling investigation of deinstitutionalization and the movement to build Community Mental Health Centers (CMHCs), the federal government "seemed oblivious" to the states' struggles. In 1967, Congress passed H.R. 6431, which renewed and extended CMHC construction and staffing grants for three more years and approved a budget for community mental health without in any way modifying the prerequisites states would need to follow to win these funds. According to Engel, "It had now been four years since the passage of the initial legislation, time enough for any fundamental flaws in the original concept to be noted. Officially, none were."

The turn of the decade spelled the end. Maryland's conservative governor, Spiro Agnew, left his post to become Richard M. Nixon's vice president. Maryland's mental health advocates immediately started a campaign to convince the new governor, Marvin Mandel, to be a champion for mental health funding, with the hope that Maryland could push for a model in which the state—not local governments—would take on the entire burden of financing the network of local community clinics. Mandel was sympathetic, and he pushed state lawmakers for more money. But it wasn't enough. The total Department of Mental Hygiene budget for 1969 was over $56 million, but ninety-seven cents of every dollar spent on mental health was still going to the hospitals. Leaving only 3 percent allocated to the community programs. The goal had been for community mental health programs to take the place of the large psychiatric hospitals. The seams were coming undone.

When President Nixon stepped into office, he examined poverty programs, the Community Mental Health Centers Act, and many of the Great Society programs that had defined the Johnson administration. He wanted evidence that they were actually working. He wanted to see hard numbers. As Engel told me, "The question for him was not, 'Oh, I'm a Republican. I hate this.' It was, 'Are they working? Show me the evidence.' And if you couldn't show Nixon's White House very clear, hard evidence, then it was on the chopping block." Nixon's attention quickly turned to stagflation and the Middle East. To put it bluntly, domestic programs without committed advocates or politically valuable constituents were vulnerable. Long-term mental healthcare had long been the province of state governments, not the federal government. The Nixon administration had no interest in micromanaging local clinics and hospitals or in sustaining a payment structure, like Medicaid, in which the federal government would be on the hook for 40 to 50 percent of matching funds.

To understand these failures, one needed to look no further than Baltimore, one of the ten largest cities in the nation, where after years of talk and optimism, there was only one Community Mental Health Center in operation by 1975. That same year, in Annapolis, Maryland, lawmakers were about as genuinely committed to the cause as Washington. According to Engel, "Construction funds for 1975 were derived from a new bond bill passed by the General Assembly totaling a paltry $750,000. It seemed that the state, like the nation as a whole, had never understood the true cost of improving the lives of its mentally ill citizens."

That day in 1972 when Dr. Phillips went toe-to-toe with a commission full of lawmakers, advocates, and medical leaders, he was almost certainly seeing the writing on the wall. Friends of his family told me that he felt a particular pressure on him as the Black superintendent of the Black hospital, serving a patient population that was often going to end up back in the very communities lawmakers had long shown little commitment to. He knew what was, and wasn't, waiting there for patients who looked like him. And at a minimum, he wanted state leaders to have to contend with that.

A 1976 report by the United States General Accounting Office (GAO) studied and compared release planning and follow-up care for patients who had left Crownsville and patients who had left one of its peer, historically white hospitals, Rosewood. They found glaring inadequacies in Crownsville's aftercare resources. The office's patient tracking efforts revealed "that comprehensive needs of the patients were not identified during the release planning process" and that community health providers (with whom these patients were meant to connect upon their exit from the institution) were "irregularly" present at Crownsville's patient-release planning meetings. The office found that "no formal written referrals to community providers" were made on behalf of Crownsville patients, and that the combination of weak referrals and absent community members meant that only a fraction of the patients recommended for mental health aftercare services were even on record in local clinics. Of the forty-seven patients that they attempted to trace who had been recommended for mental health aftercare services, only eight made it to the clinic as the result of a referral. They then found that the clinics had no records or knowledge of thirty-four of the other thirty-nine patients.

On the other hand, Rosewood—the children's institution that only two decades prior fought tooth and nail to keep a handful of Crownsville children from entering its premises—arranged direct placement for its patients with local providers and offered a year's worth of follow-up and assistance in transition to other public or private facilities. Rosewood's planning meetings included representatives from the psychology department, educators, speech and hearing skill workers, and vocational counselors. Although Crownsville primarily served adults, the hospital was still home to many children seeking foster care services and young adults in need of education. But the community members listed as "irregularly" attending their planning meetings included social workers, probation officers, juvenile caseworkers, legal aides, alcoholic counselors, and representatives of the Board of Education. It appeared Crownsville's patients were not only receiving less care, but when they did get support, they were more likely to have contact with people adjacent to the criminal justice system than the kinds of professionals who would have welcomed them back into jobs and school—the fundamental pillars that form community.

In one section, the GAO researchers reflected on the broader attitudes and roadblocks facing community reform. They took note of parents of institutionalized children who wanted their kids to stay in a large hospital, who refused to visit, and who believed "deinstitutionalization to be a threat to their lifestyle." They acknowledged, however, that children with developmental differences still experienced far more compassion than the mentally ill. They observed a society that was generally "repulsed" by patients, and which was actively engaging in restrictive zoning to prevent the construction of group homes in certain neighborhoods.

Undercover in C Building

Douglas Struck, an ambitious young reporter covering cops and crime at the *Evening Capital* newspaper in Annapolis, walked over to his editor's desk with an idea. "I'm going to go undercover at Crownsville."

The two men put their heads together. They wouldn't be able to get a physician's referral for this, but they figured they could always enter the state hospital as a walk-in. So they decided to research symptoms of a mental disorder and practice an authentic reenactment of it. Depression seemed like the best choice.

So late on a Friday afternoon, Doug and his editor, both white men, walked up to Crownsville's administrative building. The editor had rehearsed his lines. "This man was my taxi driver. He's been talking about killing himself!" Doug, normally an upright and confident guy, looked downcast, determined to put on his best performance of gloom and doom.

He told the intake person all about how he was feeling lethargic. Check. I don't have an appetite. Check. I don't know if I want to be alive.

Check. Oh, I don't have much desire to do anything. Check. That was all she needed to hear. Doug was in. An hour later, he was interviewed by a doctor and driven to C Building.

"I was sort of perp-walked by three attendants up to Building C, which was a large three-story, fairly old, brick building, and up the steps," Doug recalls. At each stage of that journey, heavy steel doors would slam shut behind him. Doug was brought into one of the men's wards and deposited into a large room with linoleum floors. The room had plastic furniture off on one side and an area of beds on the other, but was otherwise bare.

Just outside the room, in the center of the ward, was a caged-in office. Doug noticed that most of the attendants spent their shift in that room, looking at the patients from a distance.

Within a few hours, one of the attendants emerged from the barred office to greet him. After introducing herself and saying hello, the woman handed Doug a cup with a yellow liquid. "Here, drink this." At this time, Doug had only spoken to one intake person in depth about what he was struggling with. He told her he didn't want to drink it. He says she told him that he didn't really have a choice. So Doug drank the weird yellow fluid while the attendant watched closely. After he returned the cup empty, she had him open his mouth to prove that he had swallowed it all. This was the routine.

Doug retreated, taking in as much as possible about his surroundings, scribbling furiously into a little notebook. He took note of the padlocked windows, metal screens, and locks he saw everywhere. The space was relatively clean, but with no ventilation, the smell of disinfectant materials constantly lingered in the air. Except for a single Ping-Pong table, Doug didn't see much for the twenty or so patients housed in the ward to do. That didn't seem to matter. Within ninety minutes, Doug realized that the yellow liquid he had just drunk was the antipsychotic Mellaril. He slumped down to the floor.

It was the mid-1970s, and journalists like Doug were starting to get a sense something was wrong at places like Crownsville, and they knew this not through patients or community members. They could see it in court. Doug would visit the courthouse every day and just go over whatever new cases had been filed. While seated on a wooden bench, Doug noticed something peculiar: petition after petition filed by public defenders for people who were in Crownsville Hospital Center. Most of these petitions were arguing for a patient's release on the grounds that they were no longer (or were never) a threat to themselves or society.

After checking the archives and asking around, Doug realized that no one seemed to be paying attention to the people being funneled into the asylum through the legal system. "Occasionally," Doug recalled, "there were little police briefs about somebody who maybe walked off from the grounds; occasionally some of them were found dead in the fields around there from exposure." The private psychiatric community was almost never sending people to Crownsville.

For the next six days, Doug lived on the ward with twenty men. He wasn't the only white guy, either. There was a mix of white and Black men, many of whom had been sent to Crownsville on court orders after having been found mentally incapacitated.

Although he didn't report it in the paper at the time, Doug recalls listening to the unmistakable sound of patients having sex at night. He watched time and again as patients who he sensed craved human interaction approached the bars of the staff's cage. The aides yelled at them to go away.

Three times a day, men and women housed all over the building gathered in one massive dining hall. To him, it seemed there was a constant enforcement of docility, and patients were regularly threatened with solitary confinement for defying the rules. People tried very hard to resist being drugged. Some of the men became skilled at half swallowing the medication they were forced to take. When the nurse turned away, they'd vomit it up.

Occasionally, Doug watched as patients were gang-tackled by staff for being too loud or disruptive. During one meal, a patient was grabbed and swung around by her hair. He made note of patients he saw with bruises.

It didn't take long for Doug to drop all pretense of being depressed. Nobody noticed, nobody invited him to talk or engage in therapy. It seemed to Doug that attendants could not care less about what patients did with their time or whether they got better.

After a week, Doug had seen enough. As someone who voluntarily admitted himself, staff couldn't keep him at Crownsville against his will unless he was a danger to himself. After all, Crownsville, like asylums around the country, was under pressure to reduce its numbers.

On the day he was discharged, Doug met with a psychologist for the first time. This assessment was a requirement so that staff had the opportunity to challenge his request for discharge. "They weren't about to do that," Doug told me. On his last day at the hospital, Doug got the chance to explore the grounds. Walking freely around the campus after a week of looking out through dusty metal screens, he was free again. Many others couldn't say the same.

Decades later, chatting over a pandemic-era Zoom call, Doug looked visibly angry. "There was no human care and there's no humanity there, with the exception of whatever humanity the men in the wards, you know, exhibited to each other," he told me. The long history of the asylum system seemed to be weighing on him. "By the time I entered," he explained, "chains had been replaced by drugs. So the chains were still there."

"What on Earth Can We Do with All These Kids?"

As patients at Crownsville became more subject to isolation and punishment, Black Marylanders living outside of institutions experienced a different type of isolation and restraint. In several parts of the country, Black communities were starting to see early signs of gentrification. Black Annapolitans were being pushed off their land and out of their homes and moved into urban centers and public housing.

In Maryland, you can often trace the story of Black families by looking at the water. From its earliest foundations, when Annapolis was a slave port, water acted as a symbol of the racial divide. It was where slaves waited to find out their fate, and it was where the wealthy wielded power and influence to buy people.

Even during World War II, naval ships would dock in Annapolis and the midshipmen would leave the boats and head to the nearby bars or Naval Academy. But only white sailors were welcome at the academy. Black sailors often stayed aboard. Crownsville nurse Donald Williams saw this happen to his own family members. Black sailors coming into the port had two choices: either stay on the cramped boat or travel uptown closer to Clay Street, where Black people could find their own entertainment.

The lucky few who had loved ones in the area traveled to their homes for the night. Joyce and Errol Phillip told me they would invite one particular Black sailor to stay at their employee cottage on Crownsville grounds. Together they'd go down to the water to pick him up and bring him back to their home. Their cottage became his "home away from home," where this sailor could enjoy a home-cooked meal or just spend time with them.

Well into the 1960s and 1970s, Black families called the waterfront home. Rodney Barnes, the writer whose aunt was sent to Crownsville, lived with his grandmother and mother down by the water in his early years. Those working-class families lived close to one another and built a community that felt more like a tribe. The salt in the air, coastal humidity, and neighborhood barbeques all characterized home for Black Annapolitans. But you wouldn't know that by looking at those same neighborhoods today.

In the 1970s, developers and wealthy families decided that water was recreational and made for great real estate. Suddenly everything changed.

"Developers started to move in, and that waterfront property was snatched up," Rodney recalled. He watched as his friends and family dispersed. People who'd lived along the water and next door to one another for decades were being moved out to public housing on the outskirts of town with limited public services. Initially, these new public housing developments seemed fine. But when those families struggled to find jobs at places like the Naval Academy and in other parts of the service sector, opportunity kept dwindling. The public housing developments became notorious for poverty and, later, violence.

Baltimore was undergoing massive communal and demographic shifts, too, as the Civil Rights Movement reshaped the social landscape of the city. Although many white Americans accepted racial equality and integration in principle, demographic trends from the period suggest they felt differently in practice. In 1957, Baltimore's Clifton Park Junior High School had 2,023 white students and thirty-four Black students. One decade later, the same school had 2,037 Black students and twelve white students. Middle- and upper-middle-class white families abandoned the city's public schools in shocking numbers. They fled to the suburbs in thousands, and many of those suburban voters stopped voting for welfare and social programs. During that same period, Baltimore brought law enforcement officers into its urban schools for the first time. Many of the state's young, poor, and minority students were subject to police scrutiny for infractions that at any earlier time would have been handled by school administrators.

Inside Crownsville's walls, longtime employees were feeling their own forms of alienation and displacement. Thomas and Barbara Arthur, a couple whose family had devoted their lives to the Campanella building and to creating from scratch recreational programs, musicals, and camping trips for patients, started by the late 1970s feeling as though the administration viewed their work and its role in patient recovery as an afterthought or excess. Other institutions were copying and celebrating their programs, while rumors were circulating that Crownsville was on the brink of being shut down. At one point, Thomas didn't even have an office. When he wasn't with patients, Thomas would go sit in his car in the employee parking lot, filling out paperwork, planning activities, and organizing his calendar.

Barbara recalls being directed to discharge patients to community programs that "simply didn't exist." They would let patients go—handing them a one-way bus ticket downtown—and days later, she would drive home from work and see her former patients out on the road, fending for themselves.

In March 1976, Anne Arundel's county executive rode back into office promising Annapolis residents that as the county's leader, he would make

crime-fighting his first priority. Part of his strategy included the opening of a new juvenile rehabilitation center, and it would be conveniently
located in the Winterode Building of Crownsville Hospital. The county
executive was a man named Robert Pascal. He was a Republican originally from New Jersey, and he had been an all-American football player,
business owner, and gas executive. He gave this new juvenile school a
cheeky nickname: Pascal's Prison.

His criminal justice coordinator, Victor Sulin, told a reporter with
the *Evening Sun* that the program for children was "aimed at the multiple offender who is headed for crime. This will be the last local stop
before institutional care, and the kids will know this. It's one of the
things in our favor." He described how kids who break the school's rules
would be brought before judges, and how there were three central goals:
to get the students up to a fifth-grade reading level, to ensure they were
physically exhausted so that they couldn't engage in any "night-time chi-
canery," and to provide vocational training so that they could hopefully
learn skills that would help them secure jobs in the future.

Interestingly, the reporter noted, juvenile crime had actually dropped
in the county over the last two years. Officials said this reduction was
thanks to their efforts.

Sulin told readers that in designing the program, their team had
asked themselves a central question. "'What on earth can we do with
these kids?' We found we could either educate, treat, or ignore them," he
explained. "To be honest, we wanted to do all three."

The observations that Doug Struck etched into his small notebook
became a nineteen-part published series on Crownsville, asylums, and
his personal reflections. About one-quarter of the series was devoted to
Doug's personal experience at Crownsville. Those sections were full of
vivid scenes depicting what it was like to live on an adult men's ward.
The remaining parts were full of exhaustive reporting on Crownsville's
operations.

Before publishing the series of exposés, Doug met with Superintendent George Phillips to share his body of work and offer him the chance
to respond on the record. Dr. Phillips stuck to his guns. He reiterated

that, as a hospital designated for the care of Black patients, Crownsville had been systematically neglected by the state. Doug and his editors pored over budgets themselves, comparing Crownsville to other state mental hospitals in Maryland at the time. The records analysis they did confirmed that Crownsville was comparatively underfunded and suffering from severe staffing issues.

And in fairness, Doug's account was one man's weeklong snapshot of one ward in a large hospital. His reality wasn't that of Sonia King or Faye Belt, for example. But it did reflect the kind of increasing carceral pressure that Crownsville and other institutions faced at this time. Funds were dwindling. Staff members were quitting. They were being asked to make miracles happen without any substantive political will for transformation.

"That was probably the first realization I might have had that this vaunted power of the press is pretty limited," Doug told me. Beyond the expected outrage and projected intentions, nothing changed at Crownsville or other state hospitals. "I never had any cause for optimism."

A year after Doug was released from Crownsville, he was back on the courthouse beat working on new articles and leads. While sifting through petitions, Doug happened upon the names of a few men he'd lived with at the hospital. He saw the name Leon—a man who had often been friendly and open with him, close to many patients on their twenty-man ward, and always aware of what was going on. Doug had to come to terms with the fact that he was moving on with his next assignment, while Leon and others sat on that same ward.

Doug's most optimistic reflection on Crownsville was that the asylum eventually closed. "The population of the hospital just continued to drop and drop," he said, his voice trailing off. "That didn't turn out very well either."

CHAPTER 18

Irredeemable or Incurable

I believe that madness is part of all of us, all the time, that it comes and goes, waxes and wanes.

—Otto Friedrich

A TEAM OF DOCTORS, NURSES, AND ATTENDANTS HUDDLED AROUND an old, dusty television that had been carted into the adolescent ward—the kind you could still see everywhere in 1983, clunky and weighing in at almost fifty pounds. It was supposed to be their break time, but unfortunately for them, the hospital administration had other plans. Word came down from the office that staff were required to watch an instructional video on the prevention and management of violent behavior. Someone pushed a VHS tape into the player. An actor dressed as a hospital aide stepped into the frame, all in black and white. He turned to the camera and explained that the video would show them how to take down a violent patient in groups of two or four.

In the case of a two-person takedown, he said, each team member would be assigned to an arm and a leg. You must approach the patient together, take hold of your assigned side, and then spin the agitated patient around backward before carrying them to a safer place. In the case of a four-person takedown, all four team members must approach, each assigned one leg or arm. Pick the patient up, holding tight onto your assigned limb, and get them to a safer place. Simple.

Then they began their demo. The actor walked into the middle of the stage and stuck his arms out to either side like a stunned starfish. "I am the agitated patient," he helpfully pointed out. For a few awkward moments, the man in the low-budget film just stood there. The doctors were waiting. No wiggling or kicking? Oh. No punches thrown? No contraband pulled out of pockets? The staff waited for the chaos to ensue. None of them had ever met a patient who waited so patiently for their takedown. A group of two and then four actors arrived on the scene. Each time, they grabbed the starfish by their assigned limbs and carried him calmly out of frame. The staff tried to stifle their laughter.

Unbeknownst to them, with their eyes trained on the screen, a group of teenagers had snuck up behind them, intrigued by the surreal video. Rarely did patients get such a clear view of what the medical Establishment thought of them. They quietly peered around the personnel's shoulders, watching step-by-step instructions for their own confinement.

Suddenly, the staff heard the familiar sound of a metal chair hitting the floor after it took flight across the room. A second one smacked into the wall. Two more screeched across the floor. Everyone whipped around. Here we go: a teenage boy was standing there holding a chair overhead. Time to subdue the patient and put your training into action.

A voice on the loudspeaker called out Code One. Dr. Brian Sims, a fresh-faced resident trained at the University of Maryland, rushed into the room with his colleagues. First, they pushed the rest of the kids out of the adolescent dayroom, hoping no one else would feed off the boy's energy and join in the chaos. Then Dr. Sims and the nurses advanced. Life was about to imitate art.

The boy looked back at them with a knowing grin. He dropped his chair behind him and walked to the middle of the dayroom. He stuck his arms out like a stunned starfish.

As staff approached him, the patient shouted an announcement. "Whatever limb you miss, that's the one I'm gonna kick somebody with!"

Seconds before they got to him, the starfish did a 180-degree turn. He cackled as every staff member lost their grip on their assigned limb. Sure enough, the attendant who had lunged for his right leg found his fingers struck under the patient's left foot. His point had been made.

The incident was a healthy, humbling reminder for Dr. Sims. He had arrived at Crownsville having received a message that the hospital was a broken place in need of better training and expertise. And, in many ways, that was true. But training at the University of Maryland had injected in Sims a kind of hubris—the kind that made doctors like him an attractive hire and dedicated provider but also tricked him into thinking that what had worked in Maryland's prestige hospitals was the cure-all for Crownsville.

He had become the mentee of a famous Black doctor by the name of Aris T. Allen, the same doctor who helped Gertrude deliver Faye into the world in 1953. For years, Allen had operated as one of only three Black physicians in Annapolis. Dr. Allen would go door-to-door, serving Black families who, prior to the 1960s, were not allowed inside the Annapolis Medical Center. He had been Dr. Sims's personal pediatrician and later became the first African American to run for statewide office in Maryland and to chair the Republican Party. Later, his love and guidance anchored Dr. Sims through the challenges of medical school. Few Black men interested in medicine had access to mentors like him. "I went away to medical school with the idea that I'm going to be just like him," Dr. Sims told me.

The patients and junior staff quickly and kindly brought wide-eyed Dr. Sims back down to earth. "As I stepped in there, and I began to espouse my knowledge, I noticed that people began to get up and walk out," Sims said with a laugh. On his first day at Crownsville, some of the nurses and aides stayed behind to offer him a bit of advice. "Dr. Sims, wouldn't it be a lot better if you just listened and watched to see how we operate, and then critique what it is we do?" Sims quickly realized the staff at Crownsville were incredibly knowledgeable—that he had been trained at a well-resourced school while they had been making their way in the trenches.

In President Ronald Reagan's America, budgets for social programs—including education, Social Security, Medicaid, and food stamps—were

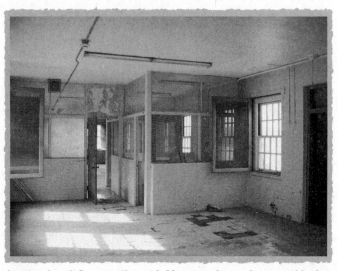

An abandoned Crownsville ward. Nurses and attendants would often lock themselves inside a protected station at the center of the room. Photo by Paul Lurz.

slashed. People were worried about drugs and panicked about urban crime. Money was flowing to the military and to prisons, jails, and new juvenile facilities. At Crownsville, the hospital was bickering with local judges constantly over who should or shouldn't be admitted there. Many involved had to laugh to keep from crying.

And on many days in the trenches there was simply nothing funny or theoretical about their work at all. Reality hit Dr. Sims hard one afternoon as he stood on the hospital's lawn, watching a police car roll down Crownsville's entrance road. Four or five officers were escorting a six-year-old Black boy, who was seated in the back in a tiny karate uniform. They yanked the six-year-old out of the car. Dr. Sims recalled the officers rambling about how the boy had been belligerent, fighting people, doing this and that. He must need mental help, they had reasoned, and they wanted Crownsville to admit him to the adolescent ward.

For a moment Dr. Sims panicked. It seemed obvious to him that the police had failed to give him the proper context. It looked like the boy had just come from a karate class, after all. But he did not want to get into it with the police, so his team agreed. "We could be held in contempt," he told me, still visibly exasperated. "And judges were very quick to do that.

If you refused [the patients] at the door, the police had no problem; they would take him back. But then they would report it to the judge and the judge would hold us in contempt." He described how Maryland judges would often issue an order and mandate that the hospital take in problem children. "It just became a fight that we knew we wouldn't win."

That afternoon, Dr. Sims and a colleague called the local judge's chambers. They did their best to professionally explain how inappropriate this was, how they shouldn't bring a child this young to a place like Crownsville. He didn't want the kid to become a victim of his fight with the court system, so even though he wanted to scream, he kept an even keel. As he made his case over the phone, the boy sat around the corner in an admissions suite in his karate outfit. In one ear, Dr. Sims listened as the judge continued to describe the boy as aggressive. But in front of him was something completely different. He was "a tiny little guy." Dr. Sims brought the boy snacks and juice; the boy said please and thank you as he waited around patiently. Eventually, the police came back to transport the boy to a meeting place with his parents.

Dr. Sims and a dozen other employees described the 1980s and 1990s as a period in which social forces outside the hospital began to closely mirror internal operations. "It stripped us of options," Sims told me. The percentage of patients involved in the criminal justice system was rising, and community support systems were shrinking away. Donald Williams, a licensed practical nurse, also recalled seeing police march new patients in and out of the hospital on a daily basis. Working in the C Building, Donald worked primarily with young Black men who he said had been abandoned or been absent from school and who, in his view, had committed thefts or assaults only after having been pushed into a corner.

Around that same time, Nick Carter, the marine whose friend, John, had died at the hospital more than a decade earlier, arrived on campus for the first time. He had been hired as a supply clerk for the state and assigned to do deliveries at Crownsville Hospital, and his sister Charlotte had become a nurse. They gave Nick keys to almost every part of the hospital, save for the wards that were locked down. At times, as he wandered around, he would think of John, and the rumors he had heard back home. "It could be scary.

Because the buildings had this atmosphere," he said. "You could hear people crying and yelling and screaming. It was something."

From 1979 to 1982 he moved into Crownsville's male dormitory building. At night, the staff would gossip about how funding was being siphoned away from the hospital. Nick became close friends with many of the hospital's aides who were working grueling, twelve-hour-long shifts. He remembers doctors and staffers calling the dorm's landline, demanding that certain aides come to the hospital during their breaks so that they could help manage or calm down the patients that they knew well. It was draining, but many of the aides had accepted that they were family—sometimes, literally—to the patients they served. When the staffing was short, Nick would see the superintendent, Dr. George McKenzie Phillips, step out on the wards and talk to the patients himself.

When temperatures would plummet in December, employees knew to make preparations for a group of patients who did not have any mental health diagnoses: homeless men and women of all racial backgrounds who would voluntarily commit themselves to Crownsville. Donald Williams described how these "patients" knew that Crownsville would always take them. For a few months they'd take part in daily life on the ward, enjoy three consistent meals a day, and play board games with other patients. Then, come Maryland's spring, they would ask to be released, preferring to live out on Annapolis's or Baltimore's streets. This certainly wasn't the first time in the hospital's history that it had become a catch-all. But after decades of staff and patient integration and investment in research, hiring of new physicians, and improvements in recreation and hospital culture, it felt like operations were sliding backward to an earlier time. A time when there were patients with no legitimate diagnosis, trapped against their will, or lost because there was simply nowhere else in Maryland to go.

Asylum to Prison

The story of America's mass incarceration and prison expansion often goes as follows: mid-century deindustrialization shatters economic opportunity in inner cities, minority communities turn to the illicit economy for work, mainstream white America fears gangbangers and crack babies and tires of the welfare state. The United States government takes a tough-on-crime stance, instituting new drug and mandatory minimum sentencing laws that disproportionately affect Black communities and lead to an influx of young Black men into overcrowded prisons. This is a powerful and thorough narrative, but it begins at its middle, not at its beginning. It does not completely address why it was that the prison—and not another social support or institution—suddenly became the chosen receptacle for America's surplus people and social ills. It was the asylum, not the prison, that had long been America's mammoth institution. In 1952, less than 150 per 100,000 people were incarcerated in state and federal prisons, while over 600 per 100,000 were living in some form of asylum. And at the close of World War II, the ethnoracial makeup of American convicts was proportional to our national demographics: approximately 70 percent of the prison population identified as white and 30 percent as "other." By the end of the twentieth century it had completely overturned to 70 percent African American and Latino and 30 percent white. Crownsville's records suggest that, while the story is nowhere near as simple as one institution morphing into the other, it is no coincidence that the end of the twentieth century marks both the decline of the mental hospital and the expansion of the prison system. And so in trying to better understand what happened to America in this period, Crownsville urges us to start the story of mass incarceration a little earlier—at a time when the prison and the asylum coexisted.

Answers may lie in the fact that after advocates successfully argued for deinstitutionalization, empathy, and community care for the mentally ill, a rise in tough-on-crime conservatism created a concurrent push to demonize and incarcerate Black people. Many Crownsville employees believed that these changes disproportionately harmed their poor and Black patients. At the very moment when wealthier white patients began to benefit from broad sympathy and private mental health resources, behaviors previously associated with mental illness led Black and poor people to be cast as criminals and, ultimately, undeserving of reintegration in their communities. In reality, it felt like deinstitutionalization didn't happen for everyone—at least, not with equal opportunity. And as a population that had effectively been twice damned and dishonored, many Black patients couldn't benefit from the open arms of deinstitutionalization's community-centric mental health mantra because they were allegedly responsible for the nation's apparent moral decline and utter lawlessness.

Historical records and employee testimony suggest Crownsville became emblematic of a broader, shape-shifting carceral ecosystem in the late twentieth century. The lines between incarceration and treatment, jail and hospital, became even muddier than they were before. As the patient became the inmate, the hospital's story raised the question: what was the difference between deeming Black populations irredeemable or incurable?

Just one month before the 1980 election, President Jimmy Carter signed the Mental Health Systems Act during a ceremony at a Community Mental Health Center in Virginia. He told the crowd gathered that afternoon that the act he was signing was "designed to provide vital services to the most underserved group in this Nation." And that it would bring some relief to the states, "which have long borne the major burden of care for chronic mental illness [and] will be able now to provide better services to all." He hoped to strengthen the dream of President John F. Kennedy—calling it the most important piece of federal mental health legislation since the JFK administration.

A few weeks later, in November, Republican Ronald Reagan defeated Carter in a landslide election. As governor of California, Reagan had been embroiled in a bitter public fight with doctors and mental health professionals after he cut the state Department of Mental Hygiene's budget. It was no surprise, then, that Carter's act found itself square on the chopping block before it ever got off the ground.

Truthfully, the entire dream of community mental health had never materialized, and it wasn't just because states had trouble matching funds and the number of centers available in major cities like Baltimore was limited. The centers had become notorious for focusing their resources on the treatment of patients who had the *least* severe diagnoses. They welcomed the elderly and adults with high-functioning depression, while those suffering with chronic and untreated illnesses like schizophrenia and bipolar disorder continued to cycle from admission to discharge in places like Crownsville. The dream died a death by a thousand different cuts. President Reagan helped close the casket and lower that dream into the grave.

On one afternoon at the end of March 1981, those choices came back to haunt him. President Reagan walked out of an event at the Hilton Hotel in Washington, D.C., when shots rang out. A man named John Hinckley tried and failed to hit the president directly, but one of his bullets ricocheted off the side of Reagan's limousine and wounded him in the left armpit. Reagan, coughing up blood, was rushed to the hospital. The man who had tried to assassinate him had been living with untreated schizophrenia and had become obsessed with the 1976 movie *Taxi Driver* and actor Jodie Foster. The film centered around a disturbed man played by Robert De Niro who plots to assassinate a presidential candidate. Hinckley had reasoned Jodie Foster might fall for him if he accomplished something similar. In the months and years that followed, Reagan remained far less interested in mental health treatment than his recent predecessors, despite having had such a close and frightening encounter.

Throughout the 1980s, national mental health advocates decried his administration's turn away from the social welfare and community interests of the sixties. Historian Anne Parsons has long studied the effect of these policies on asylums and the criminal legal system more broadly. She found that during the 1970s and 1980s dozens of developmental centers, mental hospitals, and sanatoriums were converted to prisons, and that, in some cases, the annexation of mental hospitals into penal institutions allowed states to preserve union jobs that "were important to the financial welfare" of their communities. As Parsons explained in her book *From Asylum to Prison*, conversations around mental health funding were part of a broader financial reallocation from health and welfare systems to the criminal legal system. "Politicians and policymakers worked on these issues in tandem," she argued, "as funding decisions in one realm affected funding decisions in the other and as the infrastructure of mental hospitals and prisons often guided decision-making."

The asylum became impractical in a community disinterested in institutional care for the mentally ill yet invested in the politics of crime
and punishment. According to Parsons, in the early 1980s, Pennsylvania's Republican governor Dick Thornburgh announced a crime-fighting
package to voters that included a proposal to turn Retreat State
Hospital—an asylum—into a 350-cell state correctional facility. The
conversion would cost less than building a new facility, and the prison,
which would also hold prisoners with special needs, "would eventually provide an estimated 150 jobs and an annual payroll and operating
cost of about $4 million." It reopened in 1988 as the State Correctional
Institution–Retreat. And Retreat was not the only example of an asylum being annexed into prison infrastructure. Parsons tracked down at
least sixty-nine examples across the United States of existing correctional
facilities that were once mental health institutions.

In *The Protest Psychosis*, historian Jonathan Metzl details one of the other
cases where this happened: the transition of Michigan's Ionia State Hospital for the Criminally Insane into a prison. The hospital, which initially
served a majority-white population and later experienced (and misdiagnosed) a surge of Black patients in the sixties, closed its doors in 1977.
The asylum was replaced by the Riverside Correctional Facility. Though
the institution experienced a name change and new leadership, much
remained the same.

Metzl is careful to clarify that hospitals and prisons should never be fully
equated, and yet he was struck "not by Riverside's disjuncture from the
past, but by its continuity with it." From the well-manicured landscapes to a
fully intact and repurposed administrative building, the built environment
looked almost identical. "As far as I could tell," Metzl wrote, "the only evidence of change over time—besides corrections guards mulling near the
door—were the spools upon spools of razor wire that covered the building."

The similarities went beyond the exterior. Around the time Ionia Hospital was being closed, most patients were described as "volatile African American men from Detroit." According to Metzl, Riverside's racial
demographics "clearly perpetuated those from the Ionia hospital."

271

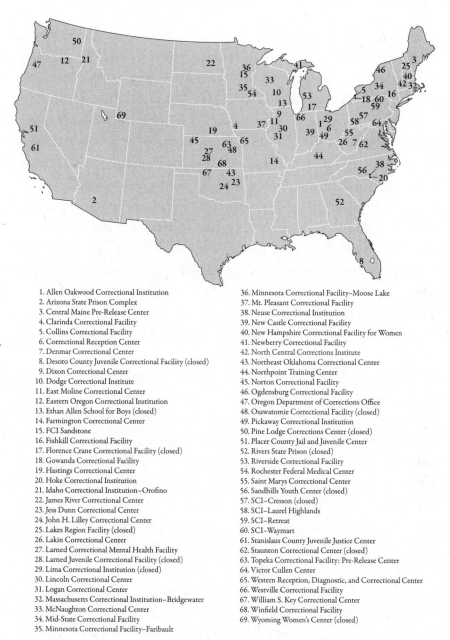

1. Allen Oakwood Correctional Institution
2. Arizona State Prison Complex
3. Central Maine Pre-Release Center
4. Clarinda Correctional Facility
5. Collins Correctional Facility
6. Correctional Reception Center
7. Denmar Correctional Center
8. Desoto County Juvenile Correctional Facility (closed)
9. Dixon Correctional Center
10. Dodge Correctional Institute
11. East Moline Correctional Center
12. Eastern Oregon Correctional Institution
13. Ethan Allen School for Boys (closed)
14. Farmington Correctional Center
15. FCI Sandstone
16. Fishkill Correctional Facility
17. Florence Crane Correctional Facility (closed)
18. Gowanda Correctional Facility
19. Hastings Correctional Center
20. Hoke Correctional Institution
21. Idaho Correctional Institution–Orofino
22. James River Correctional Center
23. Jess Dunn Correctional Center
24. John H. Lilley Correctional Center
25. Lakes Region Facility (closed)
26. Lakin Correctional Center
27. Larned Correctional Mental Health Facility
28. Larned Juvenile Correctional Facility (closed)
29. Lima Correctional Institution (closed)
30. Lincoln Correctional Center
31. Logan Correctional Center
32. Massachusetts Correctional Institution–Bridgewater
33. McNaughton Correctional Center
34. Mid-State Correctional Facility
35. Minnesota Correctional Facility–Faribault
36. Minnesota Correctional Facility–Moose Lake
37. Mt. Pleasant Correctional Facility
38. Neuse Correctional Institution
39. New Castle Correctional Facility
40. New Hampshire Correctional Facility for Women
41. Newberry Correctional Facility
42. North Central Corrections Institute
43. Northeast Oklahoma Correctional Center
44. Northpoint Training Center
45. Norton Correctional Facility
46. Ogdensburg Correctional Facility
47. Oregon Department of Corrections Office
48. Osawatomie Correctional Facility (closed)
49. Pickaway Correctional Institution
50. Pine Lodge Corrections Center (closed)
51. Placer County Jail and Juvenile Center
52. Rivers State Prison (closed)
53. Riverside Correctional Facility
54. Rochester Federal Medical Center
55. Saint Marys Correctional Center
56. Sandhills Youth Center (closed)
57. SCI–Cresson (closed)
58. SCI–Laurel Highlands
59. SCI–Retreat
60. SCI–Waymart
61. Stanislaus County Juvenile Justice Center
62. Staunton Correctional Center (closed)
63. Topeka Correctional Facility: Pre-Release Center
64. Victor Cullen Center
65. Western Reception, Diagnostic, and Correctional Center
66. Westville Correctional Facility
67. William S. Key Correctional Center
68. Winfield Correctional Facility
69. Wyoming Women's Center (closed)

U.S. Correctional Institutions Built on Sites of Former Medical and Mental Health Institutions. This map shows the locations of prisons that state governments built on the land of former developmental centers, mental hospitals, and tuberculosis sanatoria.

From Asylum to Prison: Deinstitutionalization and the Rise of Mass Incarceration after 1945 by Anne E. Parsons. Copyright © 2018 by the University of North Carolina Press. Used by permission of the publisher. www.uncpress.org

Even when prisons weren't replacing asylums, they were drawing inspiration from them. "Rehabilitation" programs and interventions focused on youth deviant behavior became a way for prisons to expand and interact with new populations. They began to copy the programs that were once found only in mental hospitals. Parsons covered the story of a prison built in Dallas, Pennsylvania—the first prison built by the Pennsylvania Bureau of Correction in over two decades. "Dallas became a hybrid mental health/penal facility and held people labeled as having mental defects and criminal propensities," Parsons explained. She found that those deemed "defective delinquents" were disproportionately African American. Parsons wrote that the construction of the facility "demonstrated the state's increased attention to law-breaking, especially among African American young people, and the inclusion of mental health in its crime-fighting."

Soon, Nick Carter found himself stuck in the gray area between illness and crime, rehabilitation and punishment. For years, he rose in the ranks at Crownsville, and graduated from a job doing physical supply deliveries to a desk job controlling state inventory. But when his sister Charlotte and brother Thomas both died from sickle cell disease within five years of each other in the 1980s, Nick felt less connected to being alive. He fell into something that was less like the dark depression he'd seen take hold of his childhood friend John, and more like a rupture. An unhinging. A former friend introduced him to crack cocaine in 1988, and feeling indifferent, Nick gave it a try. Within four years, the drug had taken everything, including his marriage and his career.

When he looks back, he realizes his grief had manifested as anger. "I was thinking, 'Why is everybody dying?'" he told me. He had seen neighbors perish from AIDS and then watched two siblings die from sickle cell, two diseases that were disproportionately harming Black people and, at the time, there was no cure in sight. Nick felt like his community had just reached new heights in their professions and influence in Maryland, only for illness, gentrification, and drugs to snatch it all back. Crack offered an escape. The high, he told me, "would take you from the top of the mountain to the very depths of life."

Nick would disappear for two or three days at a time. He would sleep in abandoned buildings or out on the street. Over the course of a decade, his family staged three interventions. "I was afraid that they were gonna try to get me committed somewhere," he told me one afternoon.

"You mean to a place like Crownsville?"

"Yeah."

Nick has been sober now for more than two decades. But he's still frustrated. "Very few Black people trust the system," he told me one afternoon. "It seemed like it's geared toward failure." He described how men like him who acted erratically or drank too much would interact with the police, and how difficult it was to have the right insurance or to afford treatment even when it was offered. His friends landed on the street or behind bars. "But let it be a white person. The first thing is, 'Oh, he's having a mental issue. We got to get him some help.'"

It wasn't a doctor or a stint in jail that inspired Nick to begin recovery. The day after the Baltimore Ravens won their first Super Bowl in 2001, he was standing on a corner getting pelted by a hailstorm. He called friends all around Annapolis to see if anyone would take him in for the night. One friend after another said no. As he stood on the street shivering, he realized, "I felt like a leper, and I wasn't wanted." He called his family and joined a rehabilitation program the next day. Today, Nick works as a chef. He spends most of his time with his four kids, twenty-two grandkids, and nine great-grandkids. Despite everything that he's been through, he's one of the few kids from his block on the Old Fourth Ward who has lived to see his seventies.

Playing Games

Paul Lurz got a call from Crownsville's chief psychologist: "You and I need to head down to the adolescent ward. There's a patient case we need to investigate." It was early 1977 and he had just received a promotion to become chief of social services. He cherished his time spent with the hospital's youngest patients, even when the circumstances were difficult. Increasingly, the hours in his workday had taken him away from the kids and clogged his calendar with meetings, hearings, investigations, and administrative duties.

Paul arrived on the ward to find a Black teenage girl locked in restraints that covered her upper body and legs. The chains on the girl's legs were so tight that she could only inch toward him by taking tiny, careful steps. She could barely lift her arms. At this point, Paul had been at Crownsville for almost two decades. Still, he was in shock. During his time on this very ward those restraints were never used.

He started asking the nurses questions and found that the ward was divided over the girl's case, and those divisions fell along racial lines. According to Paul, the teen had made remarks perceived as threatening toward a white staff member—the Black staff thought that was bullshit. A white staff member had placed the girl in the restraints for far longer than allowed by hospital guidelines and "it seemed there was no plan to end them," he told me. "This was a commonly heard complaint, that Black patients were secluded more quickly and for longer periods than whites."

Black staff told Paul in no uncertain terms that this was not happening to their white patients. He determined that this case did not stand up to a hospital review, and the girl was taken out of her chains and straps. But her release did little to ease tensions on the ward. For months, the resentment of the Black staff remained.

At Crownsville, the late twentieth century turned many of the employees' worst nightmares about deinstitutionalization into a reality. Not only was Paul shocked to find employees leaning on forms of restraint that hadn't been in widespread use in decades—he found that some of the hospital's new policies and priorities were putting patients directly at risk. For years, he'd kept a close friendship with an older patient who had a long, white beard, just like his. Paul would walk into the canteen and the patient would gesture to their matching beards and yell out, "Santa one and Santa two!"

In the mid-1980s, Paul attended one of this patient's case meetings. One of the doctors, having been pushed by state administrators to bring down the patient population, was prodding the bearded man about going home to Baltimore. To Paul, the patient seemed resistant and withdrawn. The doctor had no patience for it. "You must be afraid to leave after so many years at the hospital," he said in front of the entire group. The patient, humiliated, denied it. "I know Baltimore well and I'm not afraid. Discharge me now. I know Baltimore."

It was only a few weeks later that Paul heard the man had been found dead on the streets of Baltimore. Cause of death: hypothermia. Paul was heartbroken. "These administrative drives to deinstitutionalize [meant] that many patients ended up in night shelters if there was room and on the streets during the day," he recalled. And despite having devoted most of his life and career to the hospital, Paul felt powerless. The pressures were coming from the top down. The hospital sought to downsize at almost any cost, and in that rush, it created all kinds of hypocritical conditions. Employees noticed that some patients were being pushed out of the door directly into danger, while those who were left behind could be subject to the violence and mistreatment of a bygone era. It seemed to them that none of this represented progress or community mental healthcare.

Dr. Brian Sims continued to experience much of the same. During that period, he would work closely with patients who had been court-committed to the hospital and were fighting to get a second chance and return home. If a patient had been declared not criminally responsible for the crime that landed them in Crownsville, their only path back to community healthcare was through something called a conditional release. Crownsville staff would take the patient before a court to request that release and to negotiate an agreement about where the patient would go, how they would take medication each day, and what kind of treatment strategies they would continue to engage in. On the surface those rules sounded reasonable, but in practice it was extremely difficult for most patients to stick to them. Like an inmate on parole, patients were not allowed to miss a single appointment. These conditions would typically be in place for five years. Most people—regardless of their mental health status—could not promise to make every appointment and stick to a perfect regimen for five years straight. Inevitably, Dr. Sims would watch his patients work hard and fail anyway. "It was instantly back into the hospital. There was no pass, go, do-not-collect-your-dollars. No. You come straight back to the hospital."

What he saw was that Black patients were generally less able to afford lawyers and often at a higher risk of having their conditional release revoked. "If whites were brought in on a conditional release, it was more likely we were going to work something out. And that had nothing to do with our hospital. That had everything to do with how the courts would view it."

Maryland's institutional populations were going through immense transformations. As the state's psychiatric facilities slowly declined, the prisons accepted a record load. Maryland's Mental Hygiene Administration reported in 1976 that between 1963 and 1974, there had been a raw decrease in state psychiatric facilities from 8,100 to 5,000 residents and that the department had initiated additional programs to accelerate deinstitutionalization. In a similar period, from 1965 to 1975, the nation's inpatient population in state and county mental hospitals plummeted 59.3 percent, and by 1980, inpatient populations in asylums had declined an additional 28.9 percent.

Maryland and the nation's prisons were beginning to experience the reverse effect: the population in Maryland prisons tripled in the late twentieth century, with a raw increase from 7,731 people incarcerated in 1979 to 24,186 in 2003. By the 1990s, the United States reached a rate of opening one new prison or jail every single week to accommodate its growing carceral population. This is not to say every patient was transferred over to prisons and jails. For most of the twentieth century, state mental hospital patients were majority middle-aged and white, and our modern incarcerated populations are now predominantly young and nonwhite. It is precisely the fact that our incarcerated populations look closer to Crownsville's demographics that led me and other journalists and historians to raise questions about who benefited from deinstitutionalization and who did not. Is it a coincidence that at the very historical moment when the asylum was being dismantled, the prison, which had collaborated and exchanged extensively with hospitals like Crownsville, rose to prominence? And how might the prison have relied materially and operationally on the asylum's legacy?

What we find in Maryland is that Black men shouldered the burden of the state's prison growth: African Americans constituted 75 percent of Maryland's prison growth in the mid to late twentieth century, according to the Justice Policy Institute. Rates of imprisonment have begun to decline in recent years, but they continue to disproportionately harm Black communities in Baltimore and the Eastern Shore. When I reached out to Maryland's Department of Health and Mental Hygiene, the office that was once responsible for Crownsville's operations, they declined to speak with me or answer written questions. But Maryland's governor Wes Moore acknowledged that we have too many people with behavioral health challenges behind bars, and that "it's hard to quantify all of the ways in which America's history of racism and segregation continues to harm our communities." He had made his own inferences as a Black kid in 1982, when his father died from a rare but treatable virus called acute epiglottitis. "I know firsthand what happens when people are treated differently in our medical system," he told me. "I watched my father die when I was just three years old because he didn't receive the treatment that he needed. Instead, our family was met with questions like, 'Is he prone to exaggeration?'"

In the flamingo-pink painted lobby of Crownsville's administration building in 1983, Matt Seiden, a reporter from the *Baltimore Sun*, came across a clipping tacked onto a bulletin board that read, "Sachs Proposes Mental Hospitals Be Phased Out." Stephen H. Sachs, the state attorney general, had called for "old fortresses" to close down once and for all by the year 2000, and made the familiar promise that a network of some kind would take their place. At that point, staff weren't buying it. It had been twenty years since JFK signed the Community Mental Health Act of 1963 and promised the same thing. Year after year, Crownsville employees watched as their patient population waited for someone— anyone—to welcome them with open arms.

"Sachs talks about community facilities," Jerry Kowaleski, a Crownsville psychologist, told the *Baltimore Sun*. "But look at the realities. We've

got a long waiting list of patients who are ready to move into community facilities now, but there aren't enough community facilities out there,
and the truth is we seem to have reached the limit of what people are
willing to accept in their communities. Everyone says, 'Community
mental health centers are great'—as long as they are in somebody else's
community."

Nick Moutsos, director of Crownsville's Geriatric Division, had this
to say to the attorney general: "To say 'send them back to the community'
is pretty words, but what community? I've got forty-one people who have
been screened and chosen to go back to the 'community,' and they were
promised places and they've been sitting here for a year or more and not
one of them has gone yet. It would be a miracle if they would take even
one."

He had come to a harsh conclusion. "The only time the problems of
these people will finish is when they go under the grave. I am sorry to say
this, but it is the truth and we shouldn't play games with their lives."

In only half a century, the United States achieved arguably the greatest and swiftest institutional shift in history, at once making the mental
hospital redundant and law enforcement and incarceration of astonishing
prevalence. It is shortsighted to understand this transformation as a sudden product; as Crownsville's history shows, it was a slow, complex, and
deeply painful transition. And at the center of the societal negotiations that
reshaped our hospitals, prisons, and jails lies the Black patient. Through the
stories of employees and patients like those at Crownsville, we can trace the
desertion of the first institution and the development of the second. Black
patients and inmates served as the linchpin between these two institutions
that were collaborating and negotiating their existence in a period preceding the moment we live in now.

Love and Loss

On the night of February 8, 1991, Dr. Brian Sims got a call from a family friend. His mentor, Dr. Aris T. Allen—the man who had taken care
of him as a child and inspired him to go through medical school—was

found dead by police just before five p.m. This giant, who had been born into poverty in Texas, transformed politics and access to medical care for Black families in Annapolis, and become the chief of staff of a hospital that at one time would not have admitted him, was gone.

That afternoon, Dr. Allen had driven himself to Holy Temple Church of God and asked if he could speak to his pastor. A man at the church told him that the pastor would return soon and asked if he wished to wait. Dr. Allen waved his hand and walked back to a small rental car he'd left outside. He sat back in the car and shot himself in the church parking lot.

Within minutes, reporters arrived on the scene, snapping pictures of his car with a white bedsheet spread over the top to hide the gruesome scene. Shock and grief quickly spread through the city. Police reported that he had been diagnosed just a few days earlier with inoperable prostate cancer. All the papers wrote about how nobody could make sense of Dr. Allen ending such an improbable and generous life so violently, alone in a car. None of the papers asked whether that improbable life, which required one herculean fight after the other, might have contributed to Dr. Allen's desperation and exhaustion.

Dr. Sims has yet to make sense of losing his hero. At the time of Allen's suicide, Dr. Sims had been working with patients for over a decade and was an expert in the warning signs of depression. He took pride in his ability to provide empathetic care to Black Marylanders, whose symptoms were often misunderstood and misdiagnosed by white doctors. Somehow, his mentor had hidden his demons from him. "I was angry. I was angry because I thought that we had the kind of relationship..." Dr. Sims told me one night, his voice cracking at times. "I thought he would have said something to somebody. Talked to my dad. Even if he didn't want to talk to me, speak to them. So we at least could try to see if we could help."

About a year later in 1992, construction completed on a major traffic artery in Annapolis, a road that supports the harbor and the Annapolis Town Center. That road—Route 665—was renamed Aris T. Allen Boulevard. Even the road seemed to represent the immense sacrifice and struggle of Dr. Allen and Black Annapolitans. A decade before it opened, a different proposed path for the boulevard would have cut through a thriving Black community off of Forest Drive, and displaced many of the residents. The residents of that neighborhood had already been pushed away from the water and downtown Annapolis land. Allen had gone to the mat for them, and lobbied to ensure they were not dispossessed again.

A few years later, Dr. Sims received a last-minute call to come in and help out on an extra shift at Crownsville. He was needed in the seclusion room area. A new patient was acting erratically and belligerently. Police had picked this man up in downtown Annapolis and brought him for acute care at the hospital. Dr. Sims walked into the seclusion area, readying himself to talk to the new patient and get their backstory. He opened the door and froze.

A family member of Dr. Aris T. Allen—someone Dr. Sims had grown up with—was sitting in the corner of this quiet, bare room. On the floor with him sat a copy of Dr. Allen's autobiography. Dr. Sims and his patient and friend stared at each other for a few moments. Suddenly the patient said, "When you get a chance, you really do need to read this."

In a way, Dr. Allen has always stuck by Dr. Sims's side. His example shaped the rest of his career in the field of mental health, as a practicing psychiatrist and now as an advocate and designer of programs to improve state and federal mental health services. In the 1990s, Dr. Sims became one of the first doctors at Crownsville to introduce the practice of "trauma-informed care," a model that recognizes the importance of a patient's life story and past exposure to adverse events. It is now standard but was not common at the time. He would sit with patients and hospital aides and come up with collaborative care plans that empowered the patient to shape their own treatment and voice their worries. He encouraged other doctors to have "a plan for failure"—for what to do when their patient inevitably stumbled. Colleagues recall him as someone who found ways to innovate and act as an ally for his patients even in the face of budget cuts and policy setbacks.

In 1997, six years after he lost Dr. Allen, Brian Sims took on a new role as a conditional release monitor. It was a job typically filled by aides and nurses, since doctors usually didn't have the time to drive out into the community, visit group homes or apartments, and sit with patients who had received a conditional release. Dr. Sims loved it. He'd hop in his state-owned Dodge sedan and leave Crownsville, excited to see the faces of patients who were trying to make it through that grueling five-year parole-like system. He'd hang out with them and pepper them with questions. *How are you doing? Are you taking the medicine? Are you getting to your appointments on time? Do you need me to make any calls?* According to Dr. Sims, by the end of 1997, the recidivism rate for those patients dropped from 35–40 percent down to 5 percent.

Then he got a call. "I was just told one day that the program would be disbanded. The thinking at that time was that it was not, quote, 'an efficient use of doctors' time.'"

Not long after, he started to hear a crushing rumor in the hallways: the state wanted to close Crownsville.

CHAPTER 19

The Fire

ALMOST TWO DECADES HAD PASSED SINCE SONIA KING WALKED OUT of Crownsville's doors. She didn't imagine herself ever going back, but she did find herself thinking about the hospital all the time. She was living with her parents and her youngest sister, Deirdre, affectionately known as Dede, in a shared duplex split-level home in the town of Odenton in Anne Arundel County. Often, Sonia was the glue holding it all together. Her father was having trouble walking after suffering a stroke. Dede, who was six years younger than Sonia, was living with a developmental disability. Dede had long possessed a remarkable perceptiveness, but her ability to express herself was limited to one- or two-word sentences. Sonia had a suspicion that the passing of their youngest sibling, Marika, who arrived in the world one year after Dede, had somehow affected her sister. Marika's short life spanned a mere two months, but Sonia believed that the loss of a close companion had profoundly impacted Dede's verbal skills.

When Sonia graduated from Lincoln University, her months at Crownsville and her years spent watching over Dede convinced her that she would make a good therapeutic recreation specialist. She spent most of her waking hours devoted to others. When she wasn't helping out at home, she went to work with young people with disabilities or behavioral challenges. It was her job to welcome them to residential facilities and to develop their treatment plans or take them out on field trips throughout Maryland. She tried to remind the kids in her care of what Faye and others had always told her. *You are special. You deserve love. There is more to your story than your current circumstance.*

On Friday night, February 17, 1995, Sonia sat in the lower-level living room of her family's home reading after work. Upstairs, her father, Herbert, and her sister, Dede, were asleep. The rest of the family was out of town. Sonia heard someone call her name. The voice wasn't hysterical, it wasn't angry or even worried. It sounded like it was saying goodbye.

As Sonia climbed the stairs, she could feel heat. Something was wrong. Her father's bedroom door was open. There he was—leaned back on the bed, eyes closed and frozen still from the effects of his stroke. Flames burst around the room. Herbert had fallen asleep while smoking.

Sonia rushed forward and tried to wrap her arms around her father's legs. She tugged and tugged but couldn't pull him forward. Her hair caught on fire. She remembered looking over at the phone by her father's bed and seeing that it had been engulfed in flames, too.

Sonia sprinted down the stairs as the fire continued to spread. She grabbed the other landline phone and dialed 911. She heard a voice ask, "Fire, police, or ambulance?" Before she could reply, the line went dead.

Sonia ran and shouted. She flung herself into the neighbor's home next door. She called again. A fire truck was already on its way. Sonia doesn't think it took the fire department long to arrive, but in her memory those seconds added up to an eternity.

She shouted to the firefighters, "My father can't walk! He needs help getting out!" She tried to explain to them that her sister Dede was disabled—that they would find her in the room with the door closed next to his.

That door saved Dede's life. Sonia watched in disbelief as firefighters pulled her sister out of her bedroom window. She remembered hearing a man say, "Your father's not coming out."

Sonia and Dede were taken to the emergency room. A fire marshal came to see them. Sonia asked to see her dad.

"You don't want to see your father," the man said. "Just remember him as you saw him last."

When she returned to the house in Odenton, the home her father had worked so hard for had been destroyed. So were many of the items that might have helped her hold on to his image. What she did find were reporters swarming around the property, repeatedly asking her for comment.

For the second time, the Belt family wrapped their arms around Sonia. Faye's cousin Reverend Dr. Cynthia Belt came to see Sonia and her siblings and pray with the family. The husband of Faye's older sister Frederica prepared Sonia's father to rest through the Wm. Reese & Sons Mortuary of Annapolis. They buried Herbert King in the Crownsville Veterans Cemetery.

Sonia experienced waves of shame and depression after her father's death. I asked her how she avoided falling as low as she had in the 1970s. All she knew was that something in her was determined to avoid that depth of despair. She would tell herself that she could feel depressed, angry, and low but that she couldn't stay forever in that place. She would come close to it, but this time, she had the memory of having been there before. She told herself—this would be temporary.

Sonia also had no other choice. Dede needed her. And so did her nephew Calvin. Calvin was the son of her older sister Darnetta. His father had left him as a child, and two of his uncles had passed away, one from an aneurysm and the other from cancer. Herbert Sr. had been a father and companion to Calvin. The night of the fire, Sonia tried over and over to call Calvin and tell him what was happening to his grandfather. But he was out with friends when he looked up at a news program on television and learned that his beloved grandfather had died in a fire.

He came to see Sonia and broke down. Calvin turned to Sonia and asked her, What was the point? "I'm not going to get close to any more guys," he told her. "The guys I love only leave me." Sonia knew how dangerous it was to believe you were not worthy. She tried to tell her nephew that death was not the same as walking away. That his uncles and his grandfather loved him dearly. But Calvin was never the same from that point on.

He started drinking and experimenting with drugs. Cops would pick him up and he'd do stints in jail, where Calvin would meet doctors who would put him on medication for bipolar disorder. As soon as he got out, he would stop taking them. Odessa—Sonia's mother and Calvin's grandma—tried to love on him, but she was struggling under the weight of her own grief and anxiety. He was in his twenties, and his behavior was becoming increasingly erratic. Odessa started to worry about being at home alone with him.

Around that same time, Sonia started a new job as a therapeutic specialist for the Regional Institute for Children and Adolescents (RICA), a residential and educational facility for children in Cheltenham, Maryland. She was still traumatized by the loss of her father, and she was transitioning from working with children with developmental disabilities to focusing on teens living with emotional and behavioral diagnoses similar to Calvin's. Pouring into others when she was so depleted was hard on Sonia, but it was often a joy to be around kids.

RICA's structure and philosophy were different from Crownsville's. It was far more representative of the new model of community-based care and didn't carry with it the baggage of the historic state hospital system. The institute had specialized staff responsible for small groups of children at a time. Although part of the population came to them after brushes with the juvenile court system, it wasn't the kind of place where police could just drop someone off at the doorstep. There were interviews and screenings. There were social workers, therapists, nutritionists, and pediatricians who all had a say in the care. The residential kids had their own bedrooms and privacy—there were none of those massive, chaotic dormitories. The difference that Sonia found most startling, though, was that most of the children working with her were Black and most of the therapists and teachers were white.

Sonia wanted to be as hands-on with her children as the women at Crownsville had been with her. Sonia would try to visit her kids when, at times, they would land in the hospital. She recalled her bosses urging her not to visit her patients. She sensed that management didn't like the idea of the staff having close relationships with the students in the program.

"Just like people were there for me and looked out for me, I needed to look out for them," Sonia told me. "Because most of the people that didn't look like us didn't care." Sonia worried about how often the facility opted to prescribe medication to children. She believed medication worked and could save lives like her own. She just didn't think it was the answer for everything. Sonia wanted to avoid becoming the kind of caregiver who believed more in medication than the person.

Sonia noticed that many of her kids struggled to reach their goals and complete their work. It was not because they couldn't do it. "They wouldn't even try," she recalled. It surprised Sonia at first. She had watched children with developmental disabilities like Dede try and try again to copy what other neurotypical children could do. These kids, who were managing depression, hyperactivity, and emotional disorders, seemed to have internalized a message that they couldn't do or be anything. "A lot of what I did was try to encourage them and say, 'Hey, look, you can do this.' Life may not have been good at home. And this may happen and that may have happened." She'd tell them, "Don't get too comfortable in your room because you're not going to stay here."

As Sonia described this period of her life, I told her that it sounded to me like Crownsville had stuck in her mind. And she agreed. RICA helped her process how much community and familiarity had meant to her own recovery. A modern facility and a team with more degrees than anyone could count would only go so far. "They need to see more people who look a bit like them. People that care about them. People that have their best interests at hand," she told me. She sounded frustrated. "Yeah, it's just not like that anymore. And it is sad. I think it hinders their healing and their growth."

In 1996, Sonia observed that one of the teenagers assigned to her kept acting up the closer it got to the weekends. He lived in the residential part of the facility, where children could trade in points they earned for good behavior for an opportunity to visit family at home. He was a good kid. But as the weekend approached, his behavior would take a

Antonia Hylton

180-degree turn. He would fight and argue, refusing to cooperate. The staff would have to tell him at the last minute that he could not go home.

Sonia remembered the white teachers and staffers asking him to apologize. They would tell Sonia that what they needed to see was a sign that the boy showed remorse for what he'd done. Several weeks went by like this.

Finally, Sonia and one of the other senior therapists said to the team that if they took a look at his record, they would see that this behavior had a particular pattern over a period of several weeks. "I was like, this is a good kid! He doesn't usually do this. So something had to happen. And they were just worried that he was remorseful about what he did."

She believed something must be going on in his private life. "He's sabotaging his time to go home," she explained to them. Several of her colleagues agreed.

Sonia kept prying. Eventually the boy cracked. He had seen his best friend get killed by a drug dealer in their neighborhood. He was afraid that he and his family were next. He was jeopardizing going home because he was terrified to go home. He was willing to do whatever he needed to do to stay in RICA's facility.

Sonia was relieved to know the truth. She was also exasperated with colleagues who hadn't paid attention to such obvious signs. "They had not even considered any of that," she said.

Sonia did this work for about sixteen years. Less than a decade after her arrival at RICA, she started to hear God call her name. She trusted that she could do more good from a pulpit than she could from RICA's dorms. In May 2004, Sonia completed a master of divinity degree at the Wesley Theological Seminary in Washington, D.C. In the United Methodist tradition, Sonia committed to be sent, not to choose or to roost. She prepared for a career that would require her to travel to different congregations across Maryland.

When Sonia received her first church appointment, leadership asked her to go through a routine psychological evaluation. At the end of her intake, the counselor told Sonia they believed that she needed to address lingering anger and resentment before she could truly minister to others.

Sonia recalled the exact moment when she realized she would have no choice but to surrender to counseling. She was seated in a training session, listening to a lecturer discuss the case of a woman who had been raped. The rape had resulted in a pregnancy—just as it had for Sonia. But this woman decided to have the baby. Sonia, who has always identified as pro-choice, could feel something rise in her body as she listened. This woman, the lecturer explained, wrapped her whole life around the baby but had never taken care of herself. She killed herself.

The thing Sonia had shoved and shoved down couldn't be held in any longer. "That thing that I had stuffed way down in my toe came up to a log in my throat," she said. The tears were streaming down her face. "And it was at that point that I said, 'Okay, I got to deal with this.' And I did. I called up the resources they gave us."

She asked for a Black female therapist. Between 2005 and 2008, Sonia worked through the memories of her rape and the vision of her father in the fire. Whenever she felt she was stumbling, Sonia would call her therapist and say, "I need to come see you." She believed that her time at Crownsville made it easier for her to shed some of the stigma and to remain open to revisiting the worst moments of her life. The counselor helped her look closely at her despair and separate what had been done to her from who she was meant to be.

Sonia felt lighter. As she became an elder and an established leader in the church, she started to speak freely about her story. She hoped that it would help the congregants who came to her for counseling to find their way. But no matter what she said or how hard she tried to shower love on her nephew Calvin, he remained out of her reach.

The last time Sonia saw Calvin was in April 2021. She was living in the repaired duplex that had burned that night in 1995. She had just stepped into the shower when she heard the front door open. "Sonia!" she heard her nephew's voice bellow up the stairwell. She ran downstairs and welcomed him in. She made him a plate of food and they talked for a while.

Sonia had refused to give up on him. Earlier, she had made a few calls and found a group home willing to take Calvin in. She was feeling relieved, convinced this home was going to get him back to health. But one day a clinician at the group home called her. "Reverend King, your nephew asked me if he could go outside and smoke. And he left." When she tracked Calvin down and begged him to go back, he promised her, "I can do this on my own."

On July 5, 2022, Sonia heard a knock at the door. Detectives were standing on her steps. They showed her a picture of her nephew. Calvin had been found dead near Johns Hopkins University. They told her that he had some bad fentanyl.

Everyone in the family adored Calvin. Sonia's small grandnieces and nephews loved him dearly even though he hadn't always been around. Sonia wished there had been more they could do to heal him and to relieve some of the burden of loss and trauma. When she and I spoke in 2022, she was still coming to terms with how it all happened. She hadn't yet found the words for what they might have missed, what they could have tried—or why it was that she had found the other side of grief as Calvin slipped further into sorrow. "The hard thing is you see their potential, you know; you see what they can be," she whispered to me one morning over the phone.

A few months after Calvin's death, some of the grandchildren of her sister Darnetta were scheduled to play a soccer game. Sonia decided to see her grandnieces and nephews play. It just so happened that the game was scheduled to be played on Crownsville's old lawns.

Sonia hadn't been back since the days when she and Faye were going on their walks. As she watched the kids squeal and score only a few feet from the Meyer Building, she wondered if she should tell the little ones in her family that she had come to this place once under very different circumstances. They had understood Calvin. She imagined they would understand her story, too. But that afternoon, Sonia decided she would wait a little while. Let the kids be kids and enjoy the game.

The next day, the kids played another round of games. Sonia leaned over to her sister. "Do you remember where we are today? Does this building look familiar to you?"

Her sister looked over at the Meyer Building, with its chipping paint and shattered windows, and looked back at Sonia with a smile.

Sonia thought about the walks with Faye, the nurses who kept their eyes on her, always trying to protect her. She thought about how the love that those women had wrapped around her here had made her whole again. A love that took her years to accept. A love that she might pour into others through her ministry, her family, and advocacy.

The King sisters thanked God for where Sonia was now. When I asked her how she processed all of this, Sonia told me that she wouldn't choose a different life for herself even if she could. "The very thing that I thought would stop me was the very thing that propelled me. Because once I dealt with that, the stumbling blocks were out of the way. And I felt free."

CHAPTER 20

Closing Crownsville

Partner, Penta, and Feral Fate, two black Labs and a Belgian Malinois, stood at the foot of Crownsville's grounds, taking in a massive scent pool. The hospital's remaining 485 acres still stretch out of sight. For dogs trained to find cadavers and human tissue, this was a gold mine. "It's kind of like going into a disaster. It's a multiple-fatalities disaster so it smells everywhere," their trainer told me. At just nine months old, Feral Fate was the youngest and least experienced on the team that day. Together, the three took pause to acclimate to the powerful odor.

The area was mostly shaded early that morning, as dew clung to the grass. This was the ideal condition for the dogs to get to work. The dew helped show their trainer their path, shining the way as the herd moved through the field, and the cool temperatures kept the odors strong and localized. The morning was quiet and still. It seemed appropriate for the task ahead.

That day their job was to search what is known as the negative area—the parts of the property where historians suspected there would *not* be unmarked graves. Janice Hayes-Williams hoped that the three dogs would find a negative, remains-free space where she might place a future memorial marker dedicated to the names and stories of Crownsville patients buried on the grounds.

Since birth, these dogs were trained to recognize the smell of human blood, tissue, and bones. First, they learned to recognize simple tissue samples. Then they graduated to small cemeteries and plots. Over time, they could identify individual plots as well as the boundary of a disheveled, century-old cemetery. When they hit what they were hunting for, they performed a carefully choreographed dance for their trainer and owner, Heather Roche. They perked up, spun around, stepped over two feet, and lay down on the remains. Then they got back up, spun around again, took two steps, and lay down on the next hit. They never dug or disturbed the land. When there was nothing left to smell, they sprinted away, letting their trainer know the boundary lines.

As yellow and copper-colored leaves crunched beneath her feet that morning in November 2022, Heather Roche followed the dogs close behind to reward them for their finds, leaving markers along the pathways and banks where her little experts knew for certain there were bodies. At Crownsville, the scent landscape was a mosaic. Her suspicion was that while some of the disorganization was the fault of weather and natural erosion, much of it was the product of human disregard.

For thirty-four years, Heather has specialized in historical cadaver detection as part of Bay Area Recovery Canines (BARC) and has served as this region of Maryland's only qualified historical cadaver canine handler. She got into this strange business for one simple reason: to help people find their family members and heal. She has tried to avoid any job where her presence might do the opposite. For years, Heather was afraid to reach out to Janice Hayes-Williams and offer her assistance. On other projects, communities have asked her not to bring her dogs, wary of the history they had in some Black communities. During and after slavery, Black Americans in this area were often hunted, intimidated, and detained by patrol dogs. "It's one thing when I come out with my little black Labs that are all friendly and everything," Heather told me. It's another when she brings her big dogs.

What Heather has found is that often the dogs can sense when they've been called to a job for someone experiencing loss. Though they are not trained to be the most affectionate puppies, they will give out a spare nuzzle or come stand guard next to someone who has watched them work a site. They seem to know that what they do is important, and they can feel the difference between playful and solemn sites.

Heather, Partner, Penta, and Feral Fate searched every square inch of the Crownsville cemetery site several times over. They identified the negative space and gave Janice two options for the placement of her future memorial. In several months, their small team would return to smell through a different patch of overgrown weeds and tall grass. Janice is convinced that some of Crownsville's souls are still unaccounted for.

Crownsville Hospital Center: 1911–2004

When news broke in the local papers that the state had decided to shut Crownsville down, many of the patients had been living on the grounds for so long they couldn't imagine reinstitutionalizing somewhere new. But finding a job, safe and clean housing, and rebuilding their lives proved incredibly daunting. While there are important accounts of patients like Sonia King who successfully came home and flourished, that was not the case for hundreds, possibly thousands, of former Crownsville Hospital Center patients.

In the years after the hospital's closure, Crownsville employees found it deeply painful to travel into Baltimore or drive along Route 450 in Annapolis, where their former patients would be sleeping under bridges. Even from a distance, nurses and doctors could tell their patients had long been disconnected from their medication regimens. "Seeing so many of the patients then, you would know their faces from Crownsville. They would know you," Joyce Phillip told me, describing her daily rides along Route 450. She had worked with patients who had been at Crownsville since they were teenagers, and the hospital was all they had known in adulthood. She started to question whether deinstitutionalization had been a noble project or an abject failure and a violation of human rights. "It's hard to trust the current system that the right funding would ever be there." She believed no patient should ever be brought back into the massive, abusive warehouses she saw at the start of her career in the 1960s.

But some of Crownsville's physicians told me they estimated that up to 90 percent of the homeless people they saw in the area in the early 2000s were former Crownsville patients. There had to be a better way forward.

Rodney Barnes was still afraid to ask his family—or the government—what really happened when his aunt was sent to Crownsville in the 1970s. He didn't want to know if anyone had found her death records. While he loves Annapolis and cherishes his remaining family and friendships with people like Janice Hayes-Williams, flying home brings memories and pain to the surface. Janice, Rodney, and I gathered by Crownsville's Meyer Building to talk. Rodney was uneasy.

"When I allow myself to sort of walk around, look at the bars on the window, take it all in, there's just this feeling of sadness, you know? There's just this feeling of dreams deferred. You know, what if these people were cared for in a proper manner? What could they have been? What could they have accomplished? What would their lives have been?"

He felt that way about the entirety of the city of Annapolis. Every few months he would come back. It never got easier. To him, Annapolis represented every stolen chance and buried secret in the county. "All of it. It's like what if—what if after slavery had ended, there was truly some semblance of reparations, not necessarily the way we look at reparations now, but what if we had just gotten forty acres and a mule? What if we and our farmers had continued to own their land? What if people were able to prosper? What would our culture look like today? Instead of that, I met Crownsville and I'm at this place with these people."

Every Saturday, Rodney met with his therapist, whom he described to me as "incredibly Black." For most of his life, he resisted seeking help for persistent dark clouds of depression and anxiety. Today, therapy has made him a better friend, parent, and person. He wanted other Black men to know that it's a place to start. With a sigh, he said, "I know a lot of folks are trying to get folks to see the world differently. We could sit here all day long and talk about how poorly we've been treated as a culture. That's not what I'm talking about. How do we not duplicate the same stuff again and again and again?"

When I spent my weekends in Annapolis, Faye Belt and I would go driving and she'd show me where her patients had gone and would explain the architecture of her hometown. Annapolis, the community that looked toward the sparkling waters of the Chesapeake, had mastered the art of concealing the people, bodies, and homes it did not want you to find. But Faye knew where to look.

For the past twenty years, she had been making trips throughout the Annapolis area to check on former patients whenever she found the time. Today she runs the "Angel Network," an at-home psychiatric nurse service and hospice care company. She even offers Reiki energy healing and prayer to patients who have interest in other modalities. In between visits to her paying clients, she sometimes stops to check on the people she grew up around and treated. She keeps sandwich bags in the back of her car that she packs with long tube socks, bananas, basic toiletries, or Covid masks. The trunk of Faye's copper-brown Acura is almost always so packed, there's no visibility out of the rear window. When she can, she drives to one of two local supermarkets to check on "A" and "R," two former patients of hers who have jobs helping to return and organize shopping carts.

A lives with a loving family—Faye knows his mother well and keeps an eye on his progress through occasional calls to his relatives and from her vantage point in the parking lot. It's R she worries about.

Faye has known R since they were both young people in the 1970s, when Faye was new to nursing studies and R had recently graduated from Howard University. R identified as queer, and their religious parents, ashamed R was not heterosexual, dropped them off at Crownsville, praying for their child to become someone they were not. With their parents at a distance, R spent much of their time at the hospital experimenting with their gender. They would go down to the Campanella building and ask to shave off all of their hair, and confidently use whichever restroom suited them. When R's parents would occasionally come into Crownsville for visits, Faye remembers hearing a fuzzy mix of crying and yelling. As Faye saw it, their parents didn't realize it was they, not R, who were truly unwell. Faye believes their psychosis functions as an escape from a

Antonia Hylton

painful and unsustainable reality. R is still "in [their] safe space in [their] mind," Faye told me.

R remained in Crownsville until just before its closing in 2004, when they moved into a group home. Like many patients in group homes, R tells Faye that they are often asked by staff to leave the home during daylight hours and expected to return to a strict curfew. In recent years, investigations in Maryland and across the country have found consistent patterns of state-funded, privately run group homes that are filthy, struggling to maintain basic services, and violating safety precautions. Many of them fall back on the same restraint-heavy punitive measures that they were explicitly designed to replace. Staff are often underpaid and do not receive proper training and support. At times, patients end up deciding that homelessness is preferable to the turmoil and abuse in the homes. When she runs into patients like R, Faye grieves. She wishes Crownsville had never closed down.

The week that Crownsville's doors closed for good, Dr. Brian Sims and Faye Belt were fuming. They wanted to believe that the closure would somehow be averted or delayed by six or more months. Faye's friend and fellow nurse Gwendolyn Johnson recalled watching a group of politicians and state leaders come to tour Crownsville's wards. She took one look at them and estimated that they were 99.9 percent white. "And I looked at them . . . and I said, 'We are going to close.'"

Dr. Sims had been invited to testify before the state legislature and make the case to Maryland's lawmakers for keeping Crownsville open. These kinds of disruptions to care, he argued, especially for patients with serious diagnoses like schizophrenia, could be completely destabilizing. It could destroy trust that providers had spent years, even decades, cultivating. "Some of the families we serve do not own cars," he explained. "They won't be able to visit their loved one halfway across the state." He urged them, instead of looking to close Crownsville, to slim down and streamline all of the hospital's operations. He recommended they rename Crownsville, stop labeling it a "state hospital," and start treating it like one of the medical centers for excellence that politicians had long promised would be built. He likened the crisis of mental health to cancer, one that should be treated with urgency and staffed by dedicated specialists.

As he sat on the hearing floor, leaning forward into the microphone, patients and their families sat with a crowd in the state house, cheering him on. But this eerie gut feeling came over him as he stared back at the dispassionate legislators before him. He realized they had already made up their minds in some back room. "By the time you testify, the decision's already been made, but they just give you the time of day." They listened to him politely and thanked him for coming to the capitol.

So on June 28, 2004, Dr. Sims shook his head as buses screeched by and lined up around the campus. Administration had made their directives clear: each team was assigned a date and time when their patients were to load onto buses in an orderly fashion under the supervision of direct care workers. Approximately 80 percent of them would go to Spring Grove and the other 20 percent to Springfield Hospital. Gwendolyn Johnson's task was to help choreograph the moves of many of the patients. Several of the patients were members of her extended family, including one of her first cousins. Gwendolyn had no faith in the experiment of consolidation and deinstitutionalization. Already she had helped to discharge her family members and personally driven them back home. She would connect them to providers who said they would help her loved ones stay on medications. But it was never long before she heard they were on their way back to Crownsville. She'd ask her cousin why—and they'd tell her the community providers weren't available for appointments. "Well, half the time I can't get to see nobody!" she recalled them shouting.

Gwendolyn was there as the last patient, an older woman, boarded the final bus to leave Crownsville. Her patient seemed afraid. Gwendolyn, not knowing what else to do, lied to her and told her they were just going on a bus trip.

The doctors and nurses were expected to drive ahead of the bus to their new assigned stations at either Spring Grove or Springfield. They

would wait on the unfamiliar wards until their patients arrived. Their
job was then to smile and wave and to calm the nerves of patients who
were uncertain. Some patients' families had warned that they would be
visiting far less, unable to commute as much as two hours north. As the
patients arrived at their new hospitals that first day, they needed to see
some familiar faces. "It didn't matter what our personal feelings were,"
Dr. Sims remembered thinking. "We could have hated every moment of
it. But it isn't about us."

Faye remembers that final month in June as dizzying and heartbreaking. "Pack this stuff. Do this. Do that," was the message she remembers
receiving from interim hospital chief Sheilah Davenport and her deputies. "We left so much stuff behind," she fumed. "It was like a tornado
that came through within a couple weeks. And next thing you knew, it
was the ghost hospital."

Davenport had abruptly replaced Ron Hendler, the superintendent
of Crownsville from 1996 to 2003. Hendler had arrived to a hospital in
crisis; the state had hired thirty-three-year-old Haroon Ansari to run
Crownsville in 1994, only to discover that he had completely fabricated
his résumé. Somehow the Department of Health and Mental Hygiene
had overlooked Ansari's claim that he had run a mental health program
in Kansas City at the ripe age of thirteen. Hendler, a systems manager
with an extensive background in prison and forensic institutions, took a
tour of the campus with his wife before his first day. "This looks like a
bombed-out World War Two area instead of a hospital," she told him.

He spent the following years as leader transforming hospital operations, reorganizing staff and increasing the number of child psychiatrists,
repairing old roofs, and monitoring an effort to reduce the number of
assaults and the use of seclusion among chronic and forensic patients.
Not only had Ansari done damage to the hospital's reputation around the
state, Hendler had to navigate a patient population in which 60 percent of
people arrived through the criminal justice system. Cottage 14, one of the
small two-floor brick residential buildings at the edge of the grounds, had
set statewide records for the rate of violent incidents and staff turnover. In

exchange for all his efforts, Hendler was demoted and removed after state leaders suspected him of plotting to resist the hospital's closure.

Out on the hospital wards, complete dysfunction was out in the open. Several employees remembered seeing paperwork, including sensitive patient records, artwork, and antique wooden chairs and benches, piled up all over the place. Years earlier, the hospital administration had already thrown away a trove of crucial historical documents and patient records that predated the 1950s. They had discovered asbestos in their storage space and decided it was easier to dispose of the material than decontaminate it.

In the local papers, officials were promising the public a coordinated transition and a plan to safeguard historical artifacts. In practice, between 2003 and 2004, Paul Lurz and other staff had become accidental hospital historians and hoarders. Paul started grabbing what he could and organizing documents in fireproof containers in his own office's walk-in closet. Paul met with his friend and local archivist Rob Schoeberlein to strategize a transfer of the boxes to the state archives. Before Paul retired in April 2004, Rob would drive out to Crownsville and take digital images of records and hospital photographs. According to Paul, some records never made it to the archives, however. He was told that someone made the decision to place a collection of papers documenting past incidents of abuse at the hospital into a shredder once Paul retired from the hospital that spring.

Nurses and doctors were setting meetings with their patient groups, trying to reassure them that the havoc around them was temporary. None of them believed that, though. Morale plummeted. Staff were quietly on the hunt for new jobs, scoffing at the state's demand that they commute to new hospitals far from their homes. More than a dozen staffers were left without new job placements at all.

While the transition appeared sudden and cruel, the threads had in truth unraveled in slow motion over twenty years. The state was strapped for cash and the residential populations at all major hospitals had declined. According to state health officials and a budget proposal from

Republican governor Robert Ehrlich, Crownsville's closing would save the state $12 million.

Ron Hendler recalled seeing the writing on the wall in his final two years as superintendent. "They kept forcing me by cutting my budget to have vacant positions to cover the expenses of operating the hospital," he told me. "And then when I didn't fill the positions, they were taken from me...You know, some other department could be $20 million short and they would never have an issue. But if I was $10,000 over budget, I would get reamed out." Crownsville was the smallest of the three major state hospitals—Crownsville, Springfield, and Spring Grove—and its population had shrunk down to just over 200 patients. Half a dozen buildings were vacant while another half dozen were rented to other organizations. It was a far cry from the almost 3,000 patients living on the 1,500-acre city within a city in 1955.

What officials and local reporters sometimes failed to mention was that Crownsville had fought for years to acquire that very census cap on their population, so as to ensure that there were an adequate number of staff to work with patients. It was that cap that had allowed Dr. Sims and other physicians to start resisting the admission of some of the inappropriate involuntarily committed patients. Before then, the hospital would very often overfill—sometimes the numbers would run back up to nearly a thousand patients, as they were unable to refuse admissions. With the cap in place, finally the staff felt they had the chance to provide state-of-the-art trauma therapy and to engage effectively with patients' families, achieving the kind of results the public had long demanded Crownsville prove it could generate. While the total population went down as a result of the cap, Crownsville remained consistently close to its cap census. Once again, Crownsville employees and patients felt they had been damned if they succeeded, damned if they didn't. Somehow, following the edict of deinstitutionalization and improving the environment on the wards had earned them the distinct honor of getting shut down. In their view, the state was determined to close Crownsville.

Other employees suspected lawmakers' long-held racist beliefs about the Black patients at the hospital made it an easy target. Thomas and

Barbara Arthur believed race and politics played a role, and that the hospital "was integrated but still seen as the 'colored' place." In their view, Crownsville Hospital and the patients it served had less political power, fewer nonprofit contacts, and no pharmaceutical industry relationships. In other words, these were the easiest patients to disappoint.

Once the transition began, Faye Belt said, she was not surprised when she started to see her patients struggle to make sense of a new environment at Spring Grove Hospital. "They were treated horrible...[They went] over to a new environment, and [staff] who are there already had *their* patients there. They were overpopulated on the wards. And the patients were crying out for help." Living far from her patients and campus for once, after years of calling Crownsville home, she struggled to soothe them.

In the days leading up to the patient transfers, when asked by the *Baltimore Sun* what response she would give to patients and families frightened by the disruption, acting hospital CEO Sheilah Davenport replied, "It's something we are talking about, but we've not really come up with any good answers on this particular question." I reached out several times to Sheilah Davenport for additional comment and received no response.

A Day in the Sun

In the middle of a circular field on the far west end of Crownsville's campus stands a simple twelve-foot cross constructed of two graying slabs of wood hammered together. The cross is the only immediate indication that these grounds hold something sacred to Anne Arundel County. It is intensely quiet here, save for the sounds of catbirds and cardinals gossiping above you. I imagined Maryland's birds were surprised to see me here—we humans are only allowed on these grounds once a year. It was the early morning of April 30, 2022, and I stood here silently with Faye Belt. As she approached the cross, I realized quickly she needed space. From a few steps behind, I watched as she stretched forth her left hand. "Father God," she sighed. Her weight shifted forward, the cross supporting her.

One hundred and eleven years ago, the first twelve men came to this field in chains. As Superintendent Robert Winterode watched closely, they tested the fibers and harvested willow in the cold, before the spring ushered in new growth. The men were then marched down to Crownsville Road, where they were forced to build themselves a Hospital for the Negro Insane.

The next time patients returned to this open field, they arrived in handmade wooden coffins, carried through the trees by their fellow patients and employees. This was Crownsville's birthplace, but for 1,722 of the hospital's patients it became a final resting place.

As Faye stepped back from the cross that guards this solemn place, other Black elders from Annapolis moved forward from behind us. Many rested their hands close to the cross's heart, others kneeled down to the ground, connecting their fingers to the soil that had mixed with a century of their ancestors' bones. Some came that day because, like Faye, they had worked here and continued to feel a combination of deep pride and grief. Others came to search for stones and signs—they were hunting for their own surname, trying desperately to find the missing piece of a puzzle in their family lineage. Many of them came from families just like mine, where for years there was a refusal to talk about mental health or to acknowledge a loved one lost. Generations have kept on running, afraid to turn and look back. But you cannot outrun pain. It will creep down the branches of your family tree until it finds someone who is tiring of the sprint. It will take hold of that person who is willing to acknowledge that it is there, and demand that they find their way back through the forest.

I find myself in the forest thanks to almost two decades of Janice Hayes-Williams's unwillingness to turn away. In 2003, Ron Hendler, the second to last superintendent of Crownsville, called her uncle George Phelps out of the blue. Hendler knew the state was maneuvering to shut the hospital down and that, already, there were rumblings in Annapolis about what all this land in the heart of Anne Arundel could be turned into. He wasn't the most emotional or sentimental of men, but he knew what was at risk—what this land meant to the people he'd served. In fact, he had made his concerns about Crownsville's closing so public that he suspected Maryland's Mental Hygiene Administration would soon fire him. He made the call to George Phelps, a well-respected leader and the county's first Black law enforcement officer, and asked if he would help him clean, recover, and maintain the cemetery before someone else got their hands on it. George was stunned but quickly agreed.

Janice told her uncle George, "Whatever you doing, I'm riding shotgun." She hopped in his truck and the two rode out to the cemetery. They stepped into the unkempt field, and immediately Janice got an unsettling feeling. "Jesus Christ," George kept muttering under his breath as they walked through tall grass and over small headstones that had been tossed about. She looked over at Uncle George, a man who had seen all sorts of strange and scary things in his time as a sheriff's deputy, and noticed he looked traumatized. Uncle George had entered a sort of trance and was praying, a prayer she had heard him say many times in her life. It was what she called his "prayer for despair." A prayer that helped him find himself when it was too much to bear.

They saw flat rectangular stones scattered through the field and slipping down the side of a nearby embankment. There were few names for the people buried here, only numbers chiseled into stone, and many of them were fading from decades of erosion. At that moment she knew she had to do something. Someone or something was calling on her to match each number to a name.

Janice called around to friends and contacts at the health department. She said the staff kept giving her the runaround, constantly telling her there was no way to help her due to patient privacy laws. The hospital had locked up all the patient records. Not one to ever accept a no, Janice called Sandy Rosenberg, a delegate in the Maryland General Assembly. Rosenberg agreed to introduce a bill mandating that the state could not sell the cemetery land.

Janice realized one afternoon that all death records are public information and that Crownsville's would be no exception. She called a handful of friends and asked them to meet her at the Maryland State Archives. Over the course of the next seventeen years, Janice and a coalition called

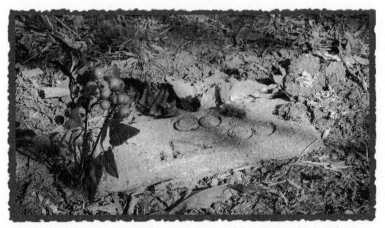

A gravestone at the Crownsville patient cemetery. Most show only a number, not a name. Photo by Christian Smooth.

Friends of the Crownsville Cemetery met up around a conference table in the archives and pored over what felt, at times, like a sea of names and numbers.

One day, not long after she started the hunt for names, she received a call from a number she didn't recognize. On the other end, a researcher from Johns Hopkins asked if he had reached Janice Hayes-Williams. "What have I done now?" she wondered. He told her that he knew she had been in the archives searching for the buried, and he wanted her to understand certain things. "You should know," she remembers him telling her, "that in the years around the Second World War the state formed an autopsy board, and every superintendent of every institution was given the power of the coroner." The man explained that any patient who did not have kin to claim their body could be sent to the major research hospitals as cadavers for medical students' training. She realized he wanted her to be ready for what she might find. "I have to tell you this journey has been gruesome," she confided in me one afternoon.

In addition to finding records for more than 1,700 patients buried in the quiet field at Crownsville, Janice estimates she has found close to 600 names of Black patients shipped as cadavers to universities. Nothing could have properly prepared her for the details in those records. Patients who drowned after running away from the hospital. A woman who died by suicide by consuming radiator antifreeze. Newborn babies. Men who had joined the Great Migration from Texas or Georgia and made it up to Baltimore, only to have their lives come to an end here.

Her team of scrappy volunteers noticed a drop in patient burials around the 1950s and 1960s. She suspected that as more Black employees arrived, fewer and fewer patients became completely disconnected from their families. "The story was out there, that this [had been] a little shop of horrors. You don't leave your family there. You don't bury your family there." Janice wondered if that was why she had heard some of the beloved Black undertakers in the Annapolis area market themselves to families in mourning by emphasizing that their loved one "would be a name and not a number."

Faye Belt and I brought folding chairs with us that day in April 2022 and took some deep breaths in the sun as we waited for Janice to begin a ceremony called Say My Name. Every year for those seventeen years, she has invited people to join her on the cemetery grounds to speak out loud the names of the patients she has confirmed were buried there. Often, only ten or fifteen people would show up. That year, hundreds came. As Faye and I waited, Delores Hawkins, Marie Gough, Joyce Phillip, Donald Williams, Barbara Shank, and many others came to join us.

It was a miracle that we were all there. Not only had Janice kept the promise she made to these burial grounds years ago with her uncle George; she had spent much of the last two decades forging unusual friendships and coalitions to protect all of Crownsville's vast property and to rehabilitate many of its most historically significant buildings. She announced that day in April that the legislature had provided an initial $30 million in funds for the county to turn the hospital grounds into a memorial, park, and museum. Janice planned to work closely on the land's development with her friend, Democratic county executive Steuart Pittman.

The two had often bickered about whose family held deeper ties in Annapolis, and as they worked on one sensitive project after another, they frequently got on each other's nerves. But like yin and yang, their personal histories opposed and mirrored each other's. His family came to Anne Arundel from Scotland in 1740, and since then, most generations have lived on the same large farm in the southern part of the county. His ancestors kept slaves and owned the soil; Janice's family came in bondage. "You want to think that your ancestors are good people, that you come from good people," Steuart once told me in jest. One of Steuart's ancestors was Dr. Richard Sprigg Steuart, a founder of Spring Grove Hospital. He was a Confederate sympathizer who opposed slavery, not because he thought Black people were equal, but because he worried it would make white people lazy. Steuart Pittman, who was once a community organizer in Chicago and has now made his collaboration with Janice a focus, sometimes sees himself in direct dialogue and confrontation with his own blood. He has made peace with the discomfort that comes with it. "I feel as though the county, just like the country, we are a microcosm, demographically and politically—that the county still needs to heal."

The previous county executives had not expressed much interest in Crownsville as a historical or community-based project. For years, developers had approached politicians to talk about turning the land into a sports stadium and commercial shopping center. Black Annapolitans were outraged. When Pittman entered office with a purple coalition of anti- and never-Trump voters in 2018, he met with Republican governor Larry Hogan. In terms of policy and ideology, there was little the two men had in common. One thing they could agree on was that Anne Arundel County should take responsibility for Crownsville.

Pittman says he saw unlimited potential for recovery and healing in the land. Soon, he and Janice recognized the road ahead was long. For decades, Crownsville's buildings had been allowed to rot: some of the floorboards had collapsed, and determined vines and the trunks of young trees had smashed through its windows. The sewage and water systems were outdated, and there was asbestos in several buildings. "It's scary for somebody in public office to take on a responsibility like that. You're saddled with it once you do it," Steuart explained. "Even if it's not clear that it makes financial sense, political sense, or any other kind of sense. It's just an obligation to take this land and turn it into something better." For what it is worth, Governor Wes Moore has pledged to help him. "Long gone are the days in Maryland where we run away from our past," Governor Moore wrote to me.

That morning, Janice set out woven willow baskets that were full of pink, yellow, red, and white rose petals and walked around the crowd holding out a bucket full of tiny papers, each containing the name of a different patient. I held on tight to the name of Frances Clayton, a woman from Baltimore who died at Crownsville on March 19, 1924, at the age of forty-one. Our crowd circled around Janice and her team of volunteers. Her good friend Scotti Preston, a singer and native Annapolitan, stepped forward and invited us all to be still and breathe in deep. When Scotti was small, her mother had struggled with alcoholism, and her grandparents committed her mother to Crownsville for treatment. That morning, Scotti launched into a song she wrote, inspired by her own memories and in honor of all the patients buried before us.

Will they ever know that I was here?
Will it ever show that I was here?
There's a memory, if somewhat faint,
And a history, it is and it ain't

There was a time above the ground when I had a past
Though I was here, we all knew it would never last
So I wonder if anyone will even care
That I was here

If you care enough to let it be known,
Then a silenced past is ready to come home
Say my name loud
Say my name clear
Say my name
So all will know I was here

Say my name loud
Say my name clear
Say my name

If it's really true that someone cares
Then it's a jubilee, feel it in the air
A day at a time
A century, too
A day in the sun
We waited for you

One by one, Janice and Scotti asked us to shout out the names of our patients. As we moved counterclockwise around the circle that morning, a voice would crack. Others would gasp for air. Someone had recognized a name.

The voice of a clergyman bellowed through the field, shaking the trees and sending birds flying overhead. We closed our eyes, pressing back our tears. "My Word tells me that they have a new name over in the Glory Land! They've got a song that even the angels can't sing."

We took Janice's rose petals in both hands and began to walk the grounds until something moved us. I wandered at Faye's side past the wooden cross to the far corners of the cemetery. We peered through the brush, down the path where, one century ago, men had pulled apart the willow plant and had been marched to their fate. Whenever a spirit called me to, I followed the lead of the elders around me. I knelt down and wrapped my knuckles around the grass and pressed my palm to feel the pulse of the earth. We placed our clusters of petals down to rest.

They've been waiting for us.

But for the Grace of God

WHEN I LEARNED ABOUT THE KILLING OF THIRTY-YEAR-OLD JOR-
dan Neely in May 2023, I was immediately reminded of my
father's cousin Maynard. But unlike Maynard, I think I had actually seen
Jordan once before when he was alive. I would come to New York City
during my summers in college, and I would crash with some of my aunts
or my grandparents. In the evenings after work I liked to walk around
Midtown and try to imagine what my postgrad life might look like in
this overwhelming city. I have a memory of pausing one humid evening
in Times Square and watching someone who looked exactly like Jordan
Neely dance, point, and smile for a crowd of wanderers just like me.

The next time I recognized Jordan Neely was on May 2, 2023, one
day after he had been choked to death by a former Marine named Daniel
Penny on a northbound F train. According to witnesses riding the subway that day, Jordan was visibly in distress. The freelance journalist who
made the infamous cell phone video of the encounter told the *New York
Times* that when Jordan stepped out in front of his fellow passengers, he
screamed out, "I don't have food, I don't have a drink, I'm fed up."

The man I saw crumpled on the floor of the train didn't look like the
young guy I had watched impersonate Michael Jackson, dressed up in
white, grooving under the city lights. This Jordan Neely looked weary
and dehydrated. His face and his clothing had aged. He allegedly

tossed his coat on the floor of the subway in anguish—but never struck or lunged toward a single person. Within moments, Daniel Penny was behind him anyway, locking him down on the ground in a martial arts hold, starving him of oxygen as fellow passengers watched and the train kept rolling on. Eleven days later, Daniel Penny was charged with second-degree manslaughter. He would plead not guilty, and his legal team would mention Jordan Neely's history of prior arrests and suggest a narrative of self-defense.

I thought of Maynard when the *New York Post* labeled Jordan Neely "unhinged" and a "vagrant" and wrote about him as though he had been the villain in the story of his own public killing. I remembered the violence and anxieties that had shaped the lives of my family members when I first learned what happened in Jordan's childhood. According to relatives, Jordan started to unravel not long after his mother was murdered by her boyfriend and her body was found stuffed into a suitcase left in the Bronx. I thought of Maynard again when I read that some of Jordan's last words were, "I don't mind going to jail and getting life in prison. I'm ready to die." Those words weren't all that different from what my father's twenty-seven-year-old cousin had shouted back in 1976, when he begged for someone to take him out of the country. They were close in age, living in different times and different parts of the country, but both in desperate need of support and kindness. They were met with almost everything but.

I called Faye Belt late one night as she was driving home from Annapolis and I asked her if and how Jordan Neely's killing had affected her. By that time, Faye and I were talking on the phone two or three times a week for this book, and she was accustomed to me calling at odd hours with heavy questions. She sounded tired and heartbroken. Faye reminded me that she had restrained countless patients at Crownsville Hospital. She'd been beaten by a veteran and she had wrestled patients in the grass. She recounted how, on one of her shifts, a female patient had randomly tried to choke her to death. For several minutes, Faye was lying on a hospital floor expecting to die. Faye had chosen this line of work and didn't expect most people to have the same stomach for it. But nothing Jordan Neely shouted on the train that day came close to what she had seen, and in her decades of work as a nurse, she had never killed another person. "Let me say this to you," she said, as she turned into her neighborhood in Shady Side, Maryland. "I was trained in all kinds of holds. We knew how to take down [violent] patients. You always leave space so people can breathe."

Faye thought it was normal for Daniel Penny and other riders to be afraid of the unpredictable. "But that young boy could've lived," she insisted. As much as Jordan Neely exhibited signs of illness, Faye believed, so did a group of people who seemed unmoved by a deadly chokehold, or who took out their phones to video someone gasping for air before they continued on their commute. Some part of their connection and humanity must have been severed, too. "Both [men] are victims of such disease," Faye told me. And yet there seemed to be less protection for one of them. "Where there is the assistance, none is available to us," she said.

Many have rightly pointed out that the police department had more than forty prior interactions with Jordan Neely, mostly for petty crimes and a handful of assaults. To them this is evidence that he posed an established and clear danger to others. As someone who has studied mental healthcare and the ways that violence and poverty push people to their breaking point, I found myself less surprised by the fact that Jordan Neely had interacted with the legal system, and more troubled by the fact that public servants had forty chances to get Jordan connected to care and had failed every single time.

Former Crownsville psychiatrist Dr. Brian Sims once described the city of Annapolis to me as the kind of place that has perfected the charming, old-world landscape in order to keep people like Daniel Penny from having to interact with someone like Jordan Neely. His city has achieved something New York and its massive, messy population and network of public transportation can't. He calls them "quiet embarrassments." Bad and painful things happen in hidden pockets and closets, allowing the city on a hill overlooking the Chesapeake to offer up half-truths about its history. There are the tourist traps where there were slave ships. Urban renewal and an aggressive campaign to preserve the city's historic

mansions have successfully transformed neighborhoods that were 80 percent Black to almost entirely white. There are paddleboards and luxury
motorboats parked where Black watermen once earned a living. "It's part
of the philosophy of Annapolis," Dr. Sims told me. "We have to find an
audience that even wants to listen. But if they do want to listen, boy, do
we have a story to tell."

The rest of us have to decide if we're open to listening or if we are
going to continue burying our heads deeper and deeper into the sand. The
crises of mental illness, housing insecurity, and income inequality bear
down on all of us. There will be more Jordan Neelys who come into public
view and refuse to be quiet about the humiliations they've endured. We
can try to construct cities and communities where these embarrassments
remain out of view, where we keep up this lie that we are separate and
unscathed, but it is only going to get harder. There are too many people
who know the truth. There are too many families with loved ones who
may call out for help in the future.

Dr. Sims believes this country needs more inpatient treatment space
and to approach mental health diagnoses the way we do cancer. Just as
we have specialists and advanced facilities devoted to specific types of
cancer, he believes we need doctors, nurses, and aides who work together
in teams focused on a specific problem of the mind. "My dream is that
you're going to equip these facilities," he told me. "You can call them
whatever you want, except state hospitals or asylums. Rename them
as what they would be: centers of excellence." He envisions a world in
which schools would train future psychiatrists and psychologists to give
patients agency and control in their care. They should stop preaching to
patients about what they should do or how they should feel, and instead
ask patients questions like, "How do you *want* to feel?" He hopes providers will partner with their patients during the development of the initial
treatment plan and be open about the fact they're going to need some
backup plans for inevitable failures. Failure, relapse, and setbacks are all
part of being human. He wants them to know it's okay to explore the
question, What if this doesn't work?

Right now, Dr. Sims worries, too many people think it is enough to keep developing new medications for diseases like bipolar disorder, depression, and psychosis and to do what they can to manage the side effects. As every clinician knows, a lack of medication didn't create the conditions for the disease. If pills are all they can offer as a profession, they aren't much of a medical profession at all. "We can't say 'Take your medicine every day and go to the clinic, and you'll be fine.' And that's not true. It is not true."

For others, like former superintendent Ron Hendler, the solution begins with the state strengthening involuntary commitment laws. These laws allow authorities to force people suffering with mental illness to enter a psychiatric facility, where providers will hold and treat the patient against their will. Politicians like Mayor Eric Adams of New York City have pointed to these laws as frontline tools to reduce homelessness and crime. Some patients will never agree to care, and the proponents of involuntary commitment believe it's impossible for our society to simply accept that those people may put themselves and others in danger.

For some families the existence of these laws is a relief. They prefer it to constant agony and uncertainty, and certainly to a jail cell. They want states like Maryland, which is one of a handful with an involuntary commitment law that does not explicitly define what "danger" means, to expand and strengthen it. Without a shared definition, judges and physicians often wait until someone is on the verge of a suicidal or homicidal act before they take action. At that point, it's often far too late to save a life.

But data tells us that not every patient is subjected to these mechanisms in the same way. For decades, Black people have been overrepresented in state mental hospital admissions, and some of their families have described harrowing and patronizing treatment. In 2009, New York released an assessment of Kendra's Law, an involuntary treatment program created in 1999 after a man living with untreated schizophrenia pushed Kendra Webdale into the path of an oncoming train. The man, Andrew Goldstein, had been turned away by providers after attempting to find help.

The 2009 report found that in the decade since the law's enactment, 34 percent of people subjected to these orders were Black, even though Black

people made up only 17 percent of the state population. Another 34 percent were white, even though they represented 61 percent of New York's
population. The researchers pointed to poverty and other urban social
factors and said they did not find evidence of racial discrimination.

Patients and their advocates haven't been so quick to absolve the state
of bias. Dr. Pat Deegan, a psychologist and disability-rights advocate,
told me it was impossible for her to let sleeping dogs lie—to ignore the
history when she looked at current conditions. "It ain't over yet. We're
still in the mire of it," she said. "People are still being routinely killed by
the police when they are having trouble out in the community. People are
still being drugged into stupors…expected to live out their lives that way.
People are still being institutionalized who are disturbing the community
and are kept there for life in subhuman conditions." She described this as
an expert and as a former patient, as someone who was diagnosed with
schizophrenia when she was only seventeen. Dr. Deegan has visited jails
and facilities across the United States. What she witnessed left her feeling like we hadn't advanced anywhere. "The human toll is remarkable."

On many nights over the phone, I've told Dr. Sims and Faye Belt about
how hopeless my family felt as we tried to get our loved one on the road
to recovery. I've also admitted to them, and to myself, that I am afraid of
what might be lying dormant in my own genetic script. How will I know
if I begin to experience these challenges someday, too? Will the people
who love me know how to help if they need to?

They've been incredibly generous. Faye sent me information about the
side effects of the medication my loved one took. She reminded me to
take care of myself, to ask for days off work, and to go see my siblings and
parents. Dr. Sims assured me my family was on the right path. "When
you're looking for answers, that's where the answer begins. When generations begin to open the dialogue," he told me over Zoom one night.
"While you may not be able to slow or stop or alter the genetics, what you
have is something more powerful as a tool. And that is earlier recognition. So that referral, and stabilization, and early intervention can take
place. And those are the only keys that we have right now."

Dr. Tami Benton, the chief psychiatrist at the Children's Hospital of Philadelphia, urged me to feel hopeful. "I've never in my career seen the level of discussion amongst so many different people about mental health," she said. She trusts that there's an appetite for change. The key will be a public health approach, she thinks, one that rewards doctors that partner with teachers, social workers, parents, and coaches to get out of the office and into neighborhoods. She would like to help teach a broader spectrum of people and professions how to recognize the signals of distress and how to intervene—the same way many of us are trained in our schools or jobs to perform the basics of first aid, CPR, or what to do in the event of a shooting or fire. "Stop making this a special superpower that mental health professionals have, because it's actually not," she argued. "The reality is, the capacity to recognize someone who is struggling and who might harm themselves is actually not hard to do if we give people the tools."

While there is so much about the biological and genetic components of these diseases that we still don't know, doctors are confident about protective and preventive factors. They are not rocket science: children need community, pride in their history and heritage, safety, green space, and open dialogue with adults that they trust. Dr. Benton believes we need to recruit more nonwhite professionals into mental health fields, and to offer them peer support as they navigate grueling and competitive educational programs. In the meantime, she tries to train clinicians who don't have a shared ethnic, linguistic, or socioeconomic background with their patients to get to know the families and their communities. For now, Dr. Benton believes the best way forward is to train a generation of healthcare providers in "cultural humility," or, in other words, the strength to acknowledge the limits of what they know and to remain open to asking new questions.

Historian Janice Hayes-Williams and County Executive Steuart Pittman are betting on Crownsville and the cemetery. Their goal is to turn the fields where patients were once put to work into a public space full of the protective factors and resources that kids and young adults desperately need. The hospital's land forms the green and wild heart at the center of Anne Arundel and greater Annapolis—a different feeling from the more manicured narrative you can find downtown. There will be public athletic fields, benches, and community events. Pittman plans to turn one of the hospital's administration buildings into a national museum that tells an unflinching history of mental health treatment. Janice is helping him recruit community members interested in serving on committees that will take on a range of responsibilities, from meeting patients and recording their stories to designing calming communal spaces. Already a food bank and a small handful of organizations treating substance abuse and behavioral disorders are operating out of old Crownsville Hospital units and former employee housing. Pittman's team is actively fielding calls from nonprofits interested in becoming future tenants, including groups that would provide housing for veterans and seniors.

One night, Janice told me that she could tell her ancestors were lifting her up. She believed that a council of elders—some of them older than this nation—were surrounding her, and that they trusted her vision. Crownsville, she says, will one day be a beacon of light and a place where people can rest, grow food, and come breathe clean air. "That is the recipe for living," she told me. "Mental health can only be helped with hope and healing of the soul. And that's the place." I asked Janice how she could be sure, and what her fight for Crownsville and the cemetery could teach the rest of the country. She laughed as she reminded me that she doesn't really know what she's doing. But for twenty years, she's kept trying to help her people anyway.

It was a reminder to me that the complexity and mystery of mental illness are no excuse to not take action, push for change, or find small ways to help the people around us. Perhaps that is part of what makes us so unsettled when we encounter others who can't conceal how sick, lost, and distraught they feel. We are confronted with a choice—when what we really want to do is to shirk responsibility. We are reminded that we are not so healthy and virtuous after all. We're forced to consider the role we might have played in isolating our neighbors, and how crazy it was that we ever thought we could alienate them, cut funding for the programs that helped them, dispose of the park benches where they might have found rest, and then somehow avoid a public confrontation. It's cruel. It's madness.

Artwork & Poetry by Crownsville Patients

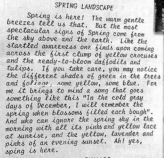

SPRING LANDSCAPE

Spring is here! The warm gentle breezes tell us that. But the most spectacular signs of Spring come from the sky above and the earth. Like the startled awareness one finds upon coming across the first clump of yellow crocuses and the ready-to-bloom daffodils and tulips. If you take care, you may notice the different shades of green in the trees and foliage, some yellow, some blue. For me it brings to mind a song that goes something like this "In the cold gray days of December, I will remember the spring when blossoms filled each bough". And who can ignore the spring sky in the morning with all its pinks and yellow lace at sunrise, and the yellow, lavender and pinks of an evening sunset. Ah! yes, sping is here.

PHYLLIS

"223"

"At 223 where we use to be. There were spirits in our home. At first their existence was unknown. But in them no one wanted to believe. More trust from each other we did need. There were spirits walking all around. Any where they could have been found.

At 223 they wouldn't let you be free. A spirit would sneak up on you quick, and they knew just who to pick. It didn't matter what you were doing. Those spirits kept on scaring. They would yell, scream, and howl; some even smelled fowl. Some had no smell at all and some smelled of perfume as I recall.

At 223 if you ever go there you might see; every turn you took, every where you looked, there was strangeness in the air. So if you ever do go there you had better be prepared to be the recipient of a scare."

Too Shy

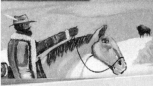

PTERODACTYL ARCHAEOPTERYX

pterodactyl, archaeopteryx
Pick up stones and pick up sticks
just a little game I play to keep
you smiling all the day.

The old man of the woods, my friend
Gorilla and his wife will never
fall, I tell you all to a man with
a sharpened knife.

ROCKY

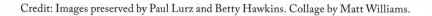

ACKNOWLEDGMENTS

This book becomes a reality with the love and help of many. I was just a teenager when I first met Evelynn M. Hammonds, Kathryn Heintzman, and Anne Harrington, the three advisers and experts in the history of science who first made me believe I could and should dig into Crownsville's story. I was so lucky to be mentored by you.

I owe a special debt of gratitude to Dr. Robert Schoeberlein for his expert fact-checking and for his decades-long commitment to the protection and preservation of the history of patients in Maryland.

Many thanks to Consuelo Hylton and Brea Baker for your edits and immense dedication, and to Mackenzie Daley and Margaret Hylton for excellent research. Cassandra Giraldo, Matt Williams, and Dave Mayers are three of the most creative people I know—they are the brains behind the artwork, maps, and photography.

Thank you to Dr. Anne Parsons of the University of North Carolina at Greensboro for your kindness when I was an undergraduate, and your support when I returned to these studies as a journalist. I also have to shout out Dr. Laurence Ralph of Princeton, who lent me books and taught me everything I know about the politics of disease and disability years ago. Thank you to Gay Hutchen for helping me navigate a tricky Institutional Review Board process.

My editor and publisher extraordinaire, Krishan Trotman, was the first person who believed all the research and hours of interviews were

222222222222

worth turning into a book. Thank you to Amina Iro and the entire powerhouse Legacy Lit team for pushing me. Maya Lewis and Tara Kennedy have done everything possible to help this book find the readers who need it. I would not have made it to the finish line without my literary agent, Johanna Castillo, and her kindness and unwavering confidence. Or without my genius lawyer, Ethan Cohan. Thank you.

Mom, Dad, Cecilia, Ellie, Norma, Consuelo, Margaret, and Keith—love you.

This book would, of course, not be possible without the patients, employees, and neighbors of Crownsville who welcomed me into their homes and trusted me with their stories, photographs, and records. Getting to know you has been one of the greatest joys of my life.

SOURCES

Part One

Chapter One: A Negro Asylum

Cartwright, Samuel A. "Report on the Diseases and Physical Peculiarities of the Negro Race." *New Orleans Medical and Surgical Journal* (1851).

"Killing Insane Principal, Most Brutal in State's History." *Baltimore Afro-American*, June 22, 1923.

Murray, Pauli, 1910-1985 and Patricia, Bell-Scott. *Song in a Weary Throat: Memoir of an American Pilgrimage* New York: Liveright Publishing Corporation, a division of W.W. Norton & Company, 2018.

Odum, Howard. *Social and Mental Traits of the Negro: Research into the Conditions of the Negro Race in Southern Towns, a Study in Race Traits, Tendencies and Prospects.* New York: Columbia University, 1910.

Schulz, Kathryn. "The Many Lives of Pauli Murray." *New Yorker*, April 10, 2017. https://www.newyorker.com/magazine/2017/04/17/the-many-lives-of-pauli-murray.

Stuckey, Zosha. "Race, Apology, and Public Memory at Maryland's Hospital for the 'Negro' Insane." *Disability Studies Quarterly* 37 (Winter 2017). https://dsq-sds.org/article/view/5392/4547.

Chapter Two: All the Superintendent's Men

Anne Arundel County. "County History." Anne Arundel County. https://www.aacounty.org/our-county/history/.

Author interview with Barbara Arthur, Thomas Arthur, Gertrude Belt, Marie Gough, Betty Hawkins, Joyce Phillip, and Thelma Lovelace. Crownsville, April 30, 2022.

Biennial Report of the Lunacy Commission December 1, 1915 to November 30, 1917 to His Excellency the Governor of Maryland. Annapolis: Press of the Advertiser Republican, 1917.

Biennial Report of the Lunacy Commission December 1, 1917 to November 30, 1919 to His Excellency the Governor of Maryland. Baltimore: Fleet-McGinley Company, 1919.

Biennial Report of the Lunacy Commission December 1, 1919 to November 30, 1921 to His Excellency the Governor of Maryland. Baltimore: Press of Day Printing Co., 1921.

Crownsville State Hospital. *History of The Crownsville State Hospital*. Crownsville, MD, 1961. Paul Lurz personal collection.

Davis, King E. "Stribling's criteria for a Black asylum." Received by Antonia Hylton, July 3, 2023.

Lurz, Paul. Letter to the Legislative Black Caucus, Maryland State Legislature, September 18, 2013.

Morgenstern, Doris. "History of the Crownsville State Hospital." Crownsville Hospital, 1960. Paul Lurz personal collection.

Proposed Outline for Ten Year (1965–74) Development Program, 1 July 1963, Reports, T2811-1. Crownsville Hospital Center, Department of Health and Mental Hygiene (General File). Maryland State Archives.

Schoeberlein, Robert William. "Mental Illness in Maryland: Public Perception, Discourse, and Treatment, from the Colonial Period to 1964." Digital Repository at the University of Maryland, May 1, 2006. https://drum.lib.umd.edu/handle/1903/3487.

The Fifteenth Report of the Lunacy Commission to His Excellency the Governor of Maryland. Baltimore: The Sun Book and Job Printing Office, 1900. http://msa .maryland.gov/megafile/msa/speccol/sc5300/sc5339/000113/013000/013150 /unrestricted/20101040e.pdf.

The Twentieth Report of the Lunacy Commission to His Excellency the Governor of Maryland. Baltimore: Press of James Young, 1905. http://msa.maryland.gov/megafile/msa /speccol/sc5300/sc5339/000113/013000/013150/unrestricted/20101045e.pdf.

The Twenty-Sixth Report of the Lunacy Commission to His Excellency the Governor of Maryland. Baltimore: 1911. https://msa.maryland.gov/megafile/msa/speccol/sc5300 /sc5339/000113/013000/013150/unrestricted/20101050e.pdf.

The Twenty-Seventh Report of the Lunacy Commission to His Excellency the Governor of Maryland. Baltimore: 1912. https://msa.maryland.gov/megafile/msa/speccol/sc5300 /sc5339/000113/013000/013150/unrestricted/20101051e.pdf.

The Twenty-Eighth Report of the Lunacy Commission to His Excellency the Governor of Maryland. Baltimore: 1913. https://msa.maryland.gov/megafile/msa/speccol/sc5300 /sc5339/000113/013000/013150/unrestricted/20101052e.pdf.

Wood, A. D. *Dr. Francis T. Stribling and Moral Medicine: Curing the Insane at Virginia's Western State Hospital, 1836–1874*. Gallileo Press, 2004.

Chapter Three: The Sea, the Farm, and the Forest

Addie Belle Admission Note, Crownsville State Hospital, March 28, 1938. Paul Lurz personal collection.

Admissions Report, Crownsville State Hospital, March 28, 1938. Paul Lurz personal collection.

Author interview with Carl Snowden. Annapolis, June 25, 2022.

Author interview with Janice Hayes-Williams. Annapolis, April 12, 2022.

Author interview with Paul Lurz. Annapolis, February 4, 2015, and February 19, 2023.

Commissioner of Mental Hygiene. Letter to Judge Thomas Waxter regarding a young Black girl in court, October 3, 1931. Paul Lurz personal collection.

"Crownsville Space Will Be Doubled: 59.2 Square Feet per Patient to Be Added Under Lane Program." *Baltimore Sun*, February 21, 1949.

Davenport, Christian. "The Roots of Reconciliation: 400 March in Annapolis to Help Heal Slavery's Wounds." *Washington Post*, September 30, 2004.

Ellis, Clifton, and Rebecca Ginsburg. *Slavery in the City: Architecture and Landscapes of Urban Slavery in North America*. Charlottesville: University of Virginia Press, 2017.

Fitzgerald, Alice. "Report of Visit of Inspection to Crownsville State Hospital." Department Of Health and Mental Hygiene Board of Nursing (General File). 1905–1971, T1572, School Reports. Maryland State Archives.

Healy, Joseph P. Undated letter from chairman of Governor's Interracial Commission to Mr. Walter Kirman. Paul Lurz personal collection.

Interim Report: The Present Status of the Criminal Insane of Maryland, 1952. S215, box 34, Department of Mental Hygiene Board of Review (General File) 1951–1961. Maryland State Archives.

Johnston, James H. *From Slave Ship to Harvard: Yarrow Mamout and the History of an African American Family*. New York: Fordham University Press, 2012.

Lurz, Paul. Letter to the Legislative Black Caucus, Maryland State Legislature, September 18, 2013. Paul Lurz personal collection.

"Meeting Minutes, March 18, 1954." S215, box 34, Department of Mental Hygiene Board of Review (General File) 1951–1961. Maryland State Archives; Crownsville State Hospital Comparative Statistics 1949–1961. 1961, box 35, Mental Hygiene Board of Review (General File) 1951–1961. Maryland State Archives.

Millward, Jessica. *Finding Charity's Folk: Enslaved and Free Black Women in Maryland*. Athens: University of Georgia Press, 2015.

"Patients Help to Build: Negroes at Crownsville Benefited by Outdoor Work. Receiving Ward Open Soon." *Baltimore Sun*, December 27, 1912.

Proposed Outline for Ten Year (1965–74) Development Program, 1 July 1963, Reports, T2811-1. Crownsville Hospital Center, Department of Health and Mental Hygiene (General File). Maryland State Archives.

Region III, Philadelphia Department of Health, Education, and Welfare and other Federal Agencies. "Deinstitutionalization of the Mentally Disabled in Maryland." United States General Accounting Office, Washington Regional Office, July 7, 1976. http://www.gao.gov/assets/200/191192.pdf.

Report on the Mental Hospitals of the State of Maryland, 1949, Reports, T2811-1. Crownsville Hospital Center, Department of Health and Mental Hygiene (General File). Maryland State Archives.

Schablitsky, Julie M. "Belvoir's Legacy." *Archaeology* 69 (November/December 2016): 55–63.

Stuckey, Zosha. "Race, Apology, and Public Memory at Maryland's Hospital for the 'Negro' Insane." *Disability Studies Quarterly* 37 (Winter 2017). https://dsq-sds.org/article/view/5392/4547.

The Fifteenth Report of the Lunacy Commission to His Excellency the Governor of Maryland. Baltimore: The Sun Book and Job Printing Office, 1900. http://msa.maryland.gov/megafile/msa/speccol/sc5300/sc5339/000113/013000/013150/unrestricted/20101040e.pdf.

The Twentieth Report of the Lunacy Commission to His Excellency the Governor of Maryland. Baltimore: The Sun Book and Job Printing Office, 1905. http://msa

.maryland.gov/megafile/msa/speccol/sc5300/sc5339/000113/013000/013150 /unrestricted/20101045e.pdf.

The Twenty-Fifth Report of the Lunacy Commission to His Excellency the Governor of Maryland. Baltimore: The Sun Book and Job Printing Office, 1910.

Weill Cornell Medical College. "The Rise and Decline of Psychiatric Hydrotherapy." Oskar Diethelm Library. http://www.cornellpsychiatry.org/history/osk_die_lib /hydrotherapy/default.htm.

Wennersten, John R. "John W. Crisfield and Civil War Politics on Maryland's Eastern Shore, 1860–1864." *Maryland Historical Magazine* 99 (Spring 2004): 5–15. https:// msa.maryland.gov/megafile/msa/speccol/sc5800/sc5881/000001/000000/000394 /pdf/msa_sc_5881_1_394.pdf.

Whitman, T. Stephen. *The Price of Freedom: Slavery and Manumission in Baltimore and Early National Maryland.* Lexington: University Press of Kentucky, 1997.

Chapter Four: What Could Drive a Black Person Mad?

Anne Arundel County. "County History." Anne Arundel County. https://www .aacounty.org/our-county/history/.

"Armwood Quit School in 5th Grade, Says Pal." *Baltimore Afro-American,* October 21, 1933.

"Badges Discussed for Crownsville: Steps Taken to Identify 'Safe' Mental Patients." *Baltimore Sun,* August 6, 1948.

Baltimore City. Grand Jury Report, May Term. "The House of Reformation for Colored Boys," 1927. Maryland State Archives. BRG68-1-5-3-2.

"Blame Ritchie in Lynching." *Washington Times,* December 5, 1931.

"Commander of State Police Gives Own Account of Attack on Jail." *Salisbury Times,* October 19, 1933.

"Comment of Eastern Shore Newspapers on Lynching." *Baltimore Sun,* December 5, 1931.

"Crownsville Issue Left to Hospital Head: Escape Problem One of Administration, Mental Hygiene Board Says." *Baltimore Sun,* August 13, 1948.

Equal Justice Initiative. "On This Day—Oct 18, 1933: White Mob of 2,000 People Lynches George Armwood in Maryland." https://calendar.eji.org/racial-injustice /oct/18.

"George Armwood (b. 1911—d. 1933)." Archives of Maryland Biographical Series, MSA SC 3520-13750. https://msa.maryland.gov/megafile/msa/speccol/sc3500 /sc3520/013750/html.

Ifill, Sherrilyn A. *On the Court-House Lawn: Confronting the Legacy of Lynching in the Twenty-First Century.* Boston: Beacon Press, 2007.

Interim Report: The Present Status of the Criminal Insane of Maryland, 1952. S215, box 34, Department of Mental Hygiene Board of Review (General File) 1951–1961. Maryland State Archives.

Leffler, Merrill. Review of *Strange Fruit: Racism and Community Life in the Chesapeake—1850 to the Present,* by John R. Wennersten. *Washington Independent Review of Books,* December 30, 2021. https://www.washingtonindependentreviewof

books.com/index.php/bookreview/strange-fruit-racism-and-community-life-in-the
-chesapeake-1850-to-the-present.

"Lynchers in Salisbury Had Right-of-Way." *Baltimore Afro-American*, December 12,
1931.

"Lynching Breaks 20-Year Record." *Baltimore Sun*, December 5, 1931.

"Matthew Williams (b. 1908—d. 1931)." Archives of Maryland Biographical Series,
MSA SC 3520-13749.

"Mob Members Knew Prey Was Feeble-Minded." *Baltimore Afro-American*, October 21,
1933.

"Mob Took Negro from Her Custody." *Baltimore Sun*, December 5, 1931.

"Negro Slays D. J. Elliott and Self." *Salisbury Times*, December 4, 1931.

Norton, Howard M. "Maryland's Shame: The Worst Story Ever Told in the Sunpapers."
Baltimore Sun, January 11, 1949.

O'Donnell, Louis J. "Guard Against Racial Outbreak at Scene of Lynching." *Baltimore
Sun*, December 6, 1931.

"Officers and Posses Hunt Somerset Woods for Negro Assailant of Aged Woman."
Salisbury Times, October 16, 1933.

"Police Squad Escorts Negro Back to Shore." *Baltimore Sun*, October 18, 1933.

"Report of Impending Mob Action Heard by Ritchie in Annapolis." *Baltimore Sun*,
October 19, 1933.

"Ritchie Orders Mob Members' Arrest; Lee Trial Deferred." *Baltimore Sun*, December
6, 1931.

"Salisbury Killer Is Hanged from Tree at Courthouse." *Baltimore Sun*, December 5, 1931.

"Shore Mob Lynches Negro." *Baltimore Sun*, October 19, 1933.

"Somerset Jury Will Be Recalled for Trial of Man on Assault Charge." *Salisbury Times*,
October 17, 1933.

Wennersten, John R. "John W. Crisfield and Civil War Politics on Maryland's Eastern
Shore, 1860–1864." *Maryland Historical Magazine* 99 (Spring 2004): 5–15. https://
msa.maryland.gov/megafile/msa/speccol/sc5800/sc5881/000001/000000/000394
/pdf/msa_sc_5881_1_394.pdf.

Wennersten, John R. *Strange Fruit: Racism and Community Life in the Chesapeake—1850
to the Present*. Washington, D.C.: New Academia Publishing, 2020.

Chapter Five: The Architecture of Injustice

Author interview with Essie Sutton. Phone, April 25, 2021.

Author interview with Faye Belt. Crownsville, May 1, 2022.

Author interview with Faye Belt and Gertrude Belt. Annapolis, April 30, 2022.

Author interview with Janice Hayes-Williams. Annapolis, April 12, 2022.

Author interview with Paul Lurz. Annapolis, February 4, 2015.

Barton, Walter E. *The History and Influence of the American Psychiatric Association*. Washington, D.C.: American Psychiatric Press, 1987.

Bourdieu, Pierre. "The Forms of Capital." In *Handbook of Theory and Research for the
Sociology of Education*, edited by John G. Richardson, 241–258. New York: Green-
wood Press, 1986.

Crownsville State Hospital Comparative Statistics 1949–1961. 1961, S215, box 35, Department of Mental Hygiene Board of Review (General File) 1951–1961. Maryland State Archives.

"Dr. Camper Would Prove His Charges: Replies to Crownsville Official on Allegations About Patients." *Baltimore Sun,* January 24, 1949.

Hospital Report, Industrial Shop Report, 1 July 1950, Reports, T2811-1. Crownsville Hospital Center, Department of Health and Mental Hygiene (General File). Maryland State Archives.

"Indifference Is Blamed: Public Attitude on Mental Hospitals Is Cited." *Baltimore Sun,* January 22, 1949.

"Industrial Therapy in Mental Hospitals." *British Medical Journal* (January 1969): 202–203. http://www.ncbi.nlm.nih.gov/pmc/articles/PMC1982065/?page=1.

Jackson, Lynette A. *Surfacing Up: Psychiatry and Social Order in Colonial Zimbabwe, 1908–1968.* Ithaca, NY: Cornell University Press, 2005.

Johnson, Walter. *Soul by Soul: Life Inside the Antebellum Slave Market.* Cambridge, MA: Harvard University Press, 1999.

Jones, Kenneth. Letter to Governor Theodore McKeldin, June 23, 1952. S215, box 34, Department of Mental Hygiene Board of Review (General File) 1951–1961. Maryland State Archives.

Keller, Richard. *Colonial Madness: Psychiatry in French North Africa.* Chicago: University of Chicago Press, 2008.

"Killing Insane Principal, Most Brutal in State's History." *Baltimore Afro-American,* June 22, 1923.

Letter to Chairmen, Senate Finance Committee, House Ways and Means Committee from John S. Shriver, 25 February 1959, S215, box 34, Department of Mental Hygiene Board of Review, General File 1951–1961, Maryland State Archives.

Long, Gretchen. *Doctoring Freedom: The Politics of African American Medical Care in Slavery and Emancipation.* Chapel Hill: University of North Carolina Press, 2012.

Lurz, Paul. Email message to author. February 21, 2015.

Lurz, Paul. Letter to the Legislative Black Caucus, Maryland State Legislature, September 18, 2013. Paul Lurz personal collection.

McCulloch, Jock. *Colonial Psychiatry and the African Mind.* Cambridge: Cambridge University Press, 1995.

Minutes of Meeting, March 18, 1954. S215, box 34, Department of Mental Hygiene Board of Review (General File) 1951–1961. Maryland State Archives.

Morgan, Jennifer L. *Laboring Women: Reproduction and Gender in New World Slavery.* Philadelphia: University of Pennsylvania Press, 2004.

Patient Medical Records, 1911–2000. Boxes 13–14, T3409. Crownsville Hospital Center, Department of Health and Mental Hygiene (Patient Master Index). Maryland State Archives.

"Patients Help to Build: Negroes at Crownsville Benefited by Outdoor Work. Receiving Ward Open Soon." *Baltimore Sun,* December 27, 1912.

Report on the Mental Hospitals of the State of Maryland, 1949, Reports, T2811-1. Crownsville Hospital Center, Department of Health and Mental Hygiene (General File). Maryland State Archives.

Sadowsky, Jonathan. *Imperial Bedlam: Institutions of Madness in Colonial Southwest Nigeria*. Berkeley: University of California Press, 1999.

Shriver, John S. Letter to the chairmen, Senate Finance Committee, House Ways and Means Committee, February 25, 1959. S215, box 34, Department of Mental Hygiene Board of Review (General File) 1951–1961. Maryland State Archives.

Stuckey, Zosha. "Race, Apology, and Public Memory at Maryland's Hospital for the 'Negro' Insane." *Disability Studies Quarterly* 37 (Winter 2017).

Swartz, Sally. "Can the Clinical Subject Speak?: Some Thoughts on Subaltern Psychology." *Theory & Psychology* 15 (2005): 505–525.

Ten Year Plan and History of CHC, 1958, Reports, T2811-1. Crownsville Hospital Center, Department of Health and Mental Hygiene (General File). Maryland State Archives.

Part Two
Chapter Six: Cousin Maynard

Author interview with Betty Williams. Phone, January 4, 2022.

Author interview with Kendal Foster. Phone, April 20, 2022.

"Gun-Wielding Man Shot Down by Officer." *Mobile Register* (Mobile, Alabama), October 28, 1976.

"Shooting Victim Said Despondent Before Incident." *Mobile Register* (Mobile, Alabama), October 29, 1976.

Chapter Seven: Black Men Are Escaping

"Badges Discussed for Crownsville: Steps Taken to Identify 'Safe' Mental Patients," *Baltimore Sun*, August 6, 1948.

"Bill To Commit Deranged Filed." *Baltimore Sun*, January 29, 1969.

Conversation between Paul Lurz, Richard Hendler, and Uria Yoder, Crownsville Hospital Campus. Transcript. December 2000.

"Crownsville Insane 'Rule,' Boehm Says: Anne Arundel Commissioner Charges 'White Glove' Treatment." *Baltimore Sun*, March 2, 1955.

"Crownsville Issue Left to Hospital Head: Escape Problem One of Administration, Mental Hygiene Board Says." *Baltimore Sun*, August 13, 1948.

"Crownsville Residents to Ask McKeldin to Move Criminals." *Baltimore Sun*, September 19, 1951.

"Crownsville Riot." *Baltimore Afro-American*, February 14, 1953.

Gordon, Kalani. "From the Archives: Crownsville State Hospital." The Darkroom: Exploring Visual Journalism from the *Baltimore Sun*. January 15, 2015. https://dark room.baltimoresun.com/2015/01/crownsville-state-hospital/#1.

"Hodge Taken from a Cell to Hospital: Ex-Illinois Auditor Is Shaken After Pleading Guilty to Fraud." *Baltimore Sun*, August 14, 1956.

Palmer, Brian, Sam Weber, and Connie Kargbo. "Maryland Reckons with a Violent, Racist Past." PBS, June 19, 2021. https://www.pbs.org/newshour/show/maryland -reckons-with-a-violent-racist-past.

"Plan to Put Prison Camp at Crownsville Questioned." *Baltimore Sun*, June 21, 1961.

"Riot at Asylum: Used Gas." Brisbane (Australia) *Courier-Mail*, February 9, 1953.

"Third Uprising at Crownsville Erupts Thursday." *Baltimore Afro-American*, February 26, 1955.

Wacquant, Loïc. "From Slavery to Mass Incarceration: Rethinking the 'Race Question' in the US." *New Left Review* 13 (2002): 41–60.

Wallace, Weldon. "Crownsville Shows Gains, But It Still Has Far to Go." *Baltimore Sun*, June 1, 1953.

Yoder, Uria. Letters to Antonia Hylton. "Crownsville Hospital," June 2023.

Chapter Eight: A Burning House

Author interview with Doris Morgenstern Wachsler. Virtual, January 10, 2021.

Author interview with Dorothea McCullers and Gertrude Belt. Crownsville, February 19, 2023.

Author interview with Dr. Jim Ballard. Crownsville, February 19, 2023.

Author interview with Faye Belt and Gertrude Belt. Annapolis, April 30, 2022.

Author interview with Milton Kent. Virtual, January 13, 2022.

Author interview with Paul Lurz. Annapolis, June 26, 2022.

Author interview with Thomas and Barbara Arthur. Virtual, April 20, 2022.

Crownsville State Hospital Comparative Statistics 1949–1961. 1961, S215, box 35, Department of Mental Hygiene Board of Review (General File) 1951–1961, Maryland State Archives.

Declarations of Intention for Citizenship, 1/19/1842–10/29/1959. National Archives at Philadelphia. NAI Number 4713410. Record Group Title: Records of District Courts of the United States, 1685–2009. Record Group Number: 21.

"Group Raps Integration of Mental Cases." *Washington Post*, January 12, 1953.

Jackson, Vanessa. "Separate and Unequal: The Legacy of Racially Segregated Psychiatric Hospitals; A Cultural Competence Training Tool." Unpublished monograph. Atlanta, Georgia, 2005. https://www.patdeegan.com/sites/default/files/files/separate _and_unequal.pdf.

Minutes of meeting, September 12, 1957. S215, box 34, Department of Mental Hygiene Board of Review (General File) 1951–1961. Maryland State Archives.

Minutes of meeting, October 20, 1960. S215, box 34, Department of Mental Hygiene Board of Review (General File) 1951–1961. Maryland State Archives.

Nuriddin, Ayah. "Psychiatric Jim Crow: Desegregation at the Crownsville State Hospital, 1948–1970." *Journal of the History of Medicine and Allied Sciences* 74 (January 2019): 85–106.

"Personally Speaking." *Hospital Topics* 31 (1953): 51–56.

Richmond, Suzanne. "Social Justice Through Medical Ethics: Dr. Jacob Morgenstern's Legacy at Crownsville State Hospital." *Generations 2009–2010.* Baltimore: Jewish Museum of Maryland, 2010.

"Summer Camp, Retreats, Field Trips & Outdoor Learning in Maryland: Camp Puh'tok." https://www.camppuhtok.com.

Sunderland, Lowell E. "Crownsville, Desegregated in 1963, Still 70% Negro." *Baltimore Sun*, May 14, 1968.

Terrell, David L., Aubrey M. Perry, and James M. Ballard II. "Vernon Wellington Sparks, Sr. (1920–2002): Obituary." *American Psychologist* 57 (October 2002): 789.

Tuerk, Isadore and Kurt Gorwitz. "Maryland's Mental Hospitals Five Years After Desegregation." Maryland Department of Mental Hygiene Statistics, May 10, 1968. Paul Lurz personal collection.

Wachsler, Doris Morgenstern. "My Father's Crownsville." *Generations 2009–2010.* Baltimore: Jewish Museum of Maryland, 2010.

Wallace, Weldon. "Crownsville Shows Gains, But It Still Has Far to Go." *Baltimore Sun,* June 1, 1953.

World War II Draft Cards (Fourth Registration) for the State of Maryland. Series M1939. National Archives at St. Louis. Record Group Title: Records of the Selective Service System. Record Group Number: 147.

Chapter Nine: A Bus Ride to Rosewood

Department of Mental Hygiene Commissioner Hospital Correspondence. January 20, 1955. Paul Lurz personal collection.

Farquhar, Roger. "House Delays Crownsville Transfer Ban." *Washington Post,* January 28, 1953.

"Group Raps Integration of Mental Cases." *Washington Post,* January 12, 1953.

Letter from Clifton T. Perkins to Mr. Blanchard Randall, Secretary of State, 20 January 1955, box 742, Department of Mental Hygiene Commissioner Hospital Correspondence 1952–1956. Maryland State Archives.

Lurz, Paul J. "An Attempt At Racial Integration Of Maryland's State Mental Hospitals—1952–1963." Self-Published, 2020. Accessed December 22, 2020.

Meeting Minutes, 11 December 1952. Department of Mental Hygiene Board of Review. Paul Lurz personal collection.

"Mental Patient Shift May Reopen Suit." *Washington Times-Herald,* December 5, 1954.

Report of the Joint Senate and House Committee to Study the State Mental Hospitals of Maryland. Annapolis: Joint Senate and House Committee to Study the State Mental Hospitals, 1949.

"State Beginning Shift from Crownsville." *Evening Sun,* December 27, 1954.

"State Sends 15 Negroes to Rosewood." *Washington Post and Times Herald,* December 28, 1954.

"Suit Delays Transfer at State School." *Washington Post,* January 19, 1953.

Part Three

Chapter Ten: Love and Broken Promises

Author interview with Julia Caridad Iglesias Cardenas. Virtual, January 21, 2023.

Author interview with Maria O'Brien. Virtual, January 21, 2023.

Chapter Eleven: Out of Sight, Out of Mind

Author interview with Betty Hawkins and Faye Belt. Faye Belt's home, Annapolis, April 20, 2022.

Author interview with Betty Hawkins, Donald Williams, and Marie Gough. Gertrude Belt's home, Annapolis, April 30, 2022.

Author interview with Faye Belt. Annapolis, February 15, 2023.

Author interview with Joyce and Errol Phillip. Virtual, April 20, 2022.

Author interview with Paul Lurz. Annapolis, February 19, 2023.

Author interview with Rodney Barnes. Virtual, December 16, 2021.

"Crowding of Youths at Crownsville Told." *Baltimore Afro-American*, February 7, 1953.

"Crownsville Space Will Be Doubled: 59.2 Square Feet per Patient to Be Added Under Lane Program." *Baltimore Sun*, February 21, 1949.

"Dr. Camper Would Prove His Charges: Replies to Crownsville Official on Allegations About Patients." *Baltimore Sun*, January 24, 1949.

"If You Ask Me: Maryland Does It Again." *Baltimore Afro-American* (1957).

"Indifference Is Blamed: Public Attitude on Mental Hospitals Is Cited." *Baltimore Sun*, January 22, 1949.

Letter from Kenneth Jones to Governor Theodore McKeldin, 23 June 1952, S215, box 34, Department of Mental Hygiene Board of Review (General File) 1951–1961, Maryland State Archives.

Letter from Paul Lurz to the Legislative Black Caucus, Maryland State Legislature. September 18, 2013. Paul Lurz personal collection.

Letter from Ralph Meng to Regina Slaughter, 3 December 1956, S215, box 35, Miscellaneous File 1957, Department of Mental Hygiene Board of Review (General File) 1951–1961, Maryland State Archives.

Lurz, Paul. "Memories." Received by Antonia Hylton, 2014.

"Maryland's Mental Hospitals Five Years After Desegregation." *Maryland Department of Mental Hygiene Statistics Newsletter* (May 10, 1968).

Parker, Jeanne Bruen. "The Social Worker's Role in the Adjustment of Foster Care Patients at Crownsville State Hospital." Master's thesis, Atlanta University, 1955.

Parsons, Anne E. "From Asylum to Prison: The Story of Lincoln, Illinois." *Journal of Illinois History* 15 (Winter 2011): 242–260.

Report on the Mental Hospitals of the State of Maryland, 1949, Reports, T2811-1. Crownsville Hospital Center, Department of Health and Mental Hygiene (General File). Maryland State Archives.

Chapter Twelve: Medical and Surgical

Author interview with Betty Hawkins and Faye Belt. Faye Belt's home, Annapolis, April 20, 2022.

Author interview with Betty Hawkins, Donald Williams, and Marie Gough. Gertrude Belt's home, Annapolis, April 30, 2022.

Dr. Benjamin Rush to James Rush. *The Letters of Benjamin Rush*. Princeton: Princeton University Press, 1951.

Elsie Lacks. Certificate of Death, February 24, 1955. Maryland State Department of Health-Baltimore, copy in possession of author.

Letter from Paul Lurz to Antonia Hylton. 2014.

Letter from Paul Lurz to the Legislative Black Caucus, Maryland State Legislature. September 18, 2013.

Maryland General Assembly. *Report of the Joint Senate and House Committee to Study the State Mental Institutions*. State of Maryland. March 1949. Paul Lurz personal collection.

Minutes of meeting, February 17, 1953. S215, box 34, Department of Mental Hygiene Board of Review (General File) 1951–1961. Maryland State Archives.

Monthly Report from Crownsville. Prepared by Superintendent Charles S. Ward for Dr. Clifton T. Perkins, Commissioner for the Department of Mental Hygiene. August 5, 1957. Paul Lurz personal collection.

Nuriddin, Ayah. "Psychiatric Jim Crow: Desegregation at the Crownsville State Hospital, 1948–1970." *Journal of the History of Medicine and Allied Sciences* 74 (January 2019): 85–106.

Preston, George H. Report to Senator F. G. Stromberg. Baltimore, MD. February 7, 1949. Paul Lurz personal collection.

Skloot, Rebecca. *The Immortal Life of Henrietta Lacks*. New York: Crown, 2010.

Smith, William H. "Probe Asked of Hospital 'Gas' Rumor." *Washington Post*, May 20, 1951.

Telephone Conversation between Dr. George Preston (Commissioner of Mental Hygiene for the State of Maryland) and Elizabeth "Bettye" Murphy Phillips Moss, a reporter at the *Baltimore Afro-American* newspaper. September 13, 1943. Paul Lurz's personal collection.

Thorazine advertisement. *Mental Hospitals* 7 (1956).

Wachsler, Doris Morgenstern. "Crownsville State Hospital: A Look at Its Present and Past 1910–1960." Unpublished manuscript. 1956.

Wallace, Weldon. "Crownsville Shows Gains, But It Still Has Far to Go." *Baltimore Sun*, June 1, 1953.

Chapter Thirteen: Nurse Faye and Sonia King

Author interview with Dr. Brian Sims. Virtual, January 16, 2023.

Author interviews with Faye Belt. Annapolis, February 15, 2022; April 28 and 29, 2022; May 15, 2023.

Author interview with Sonia King. Odenton, November 18, 2022.

Author telephone interview with Paul Lurz. October 7, 2014.

Part Four

Chapter Fourteen: Screaming at the Sky

Author interview with Betty Williams. Phone, January 4, 2022.

Author interview with Keith Hylton. Virtual, July 11, 2022.

Author interview with Kendal Foster. Phone, April 20, 2022.

Caldwell, A. B., ed. *History of the American Negro and His Institutions*. Georgiaed. Atlanta, GA: A. B. Caldwell Publishing, 1917.

Cook, Eugene. "The ugly truth about the NAACP," an address by Attorney General Eugene Cook of Georgia before the 55th annual convention of the Peace Officers Association of Georgia held in Atlanta. Date unknown.

Henderson, Ray, director. *Struggles in Steel: A Story of African-American Steelworkers*, 1996. California Newsreel.

Yenser, Thomas, ed. *Who's Who in Colored America: A Biographical Dictionary of Notable Living Persons of African Descent in America*. 6th ed. Brooklyn, NY: Thomas Yenser, 1941.

Chapter Fifteen: The Curious Case of the Elkton Three

Bleiberg, Larry. "The US Highway That Helped Break Segregation." *BBC Travel*, BBC, February 9, 2023. https://www.bbc.com/travel/article/20220306-the-us -highway-that-helped-break-segregation.

"Elkton 3 Sent to Crownsville: 'OUTRAGED.'" *Baltimore Afro-American*, September 19, 1961. http://news.google.com/newspapers?nid=JkxM1axsR-IC&dat=19610919 &printsec=frontpage&hl=en.

"Elkton Three Hoped 'to Say Something to Maryland by Long Fast in Jail.'" *Baltimore Afro- American*, September 30, 1961.

"Exclusive: What Psychiatrist Said About Elkton 3." *Baltimore Afro-American*, September 30, 1961. http://news.google.com/newspapers?nid=2211&dat=19610930&id=Kdc mAAAAIBAJ&sjid=xgIGAAAAIBAJ&pg=5996,3796354.

"Juanita Nelson: Full Interview." Interviewer unknown. Archived by the Memorial Hall Museum, Deerfield, Massachusetts. http://americancenturies.mass.edu/centapp/oh /interview.do?shortName=nelson_interview.

Kennedy, Bridget. *Pathologizing Bias: Racial Disparities in the Diagnosis of Schizophrenia*. Research paper, Brandeis University Writing Program, 2022. https://www .brandeis.edu/writing-program/write-now/2021-2022/kennedy-bridget/kennedy -bridget.pdf.

Metzl, Jonathan. *The Protest Psychosis: How Schizophrenia Became a Black Disease*. Boston: Beacon, 2010.

Olbert, Charles M., Arundati Nagendra, and Benjamin Buck. "Meta-analysis of Black vs. White Racial Disparity in Schizophrenia Diagnosis in the United States: Do Structured Assessments Attenuate Racial Disparities?" *Journal of Abnormal Psychology* 127 (November 2017): 104–115.

Schwartz, Robert C., and David M. Blankenship. "Racial Disparities in Psychotic Disorder Diagnosis: A Review of Empirical Literature." *World Journal of Psychiatry* 4 (December 2014): 133–140. https://doi.org/10.5498/wjp.v4.i4.133.

Terry v. Ohio, 392 U.S. 1 (1968). https://supreme.justia.com/cases/federal/us/392/1/.

Wells, Rufus. "Elkton 3 Talk: 'Rather Die than Cooperate.'" *Baltimore Afro-American*, September 16, 1961.

Wells, Rufus. "Trio Won't Enter Pleas at Hearing." *Baltimore Afro-American*, September 9, 1961. http://news.google.com/newspapers?nid=JkxM1axsR-IC&dat=19610909 &printsec=frontpage&hl=en.

Wilson, Edmund. *The Cold War and the Income Tax: A Protest*. New York: Farrar, Straus, 1963.

Wolraich, Michael. *Blowing Smoke: Why the Right Keeps Serving Up Whack-Job Fantasies About the Plot to Euthanize Grandma, Outlaw Christmas, and Turn Junior into a Raging Homosexual*. Cambridge, MA: Da Capo Press, 2010.

Chapter Sixteen: Sympathy for Me but Not Thee

"Agent Orange: A Toxic Legacy." *Know A Vet?* https://www.knowavet.org/a-toxic -legacy-the-generational-effects-of-agent-orange/.

Author interview with Delores Hawkins. Gertrude Belt's home, Annapolis, April 30, 2022.

Author interview with Faye Belt. Annapolis, May 1, 2022.

Author interview with Paul Lurz. Annapolis, February 19, 2023.

Chow, Andrew R., and Josiah Bates. "As *Da 5 Bloods* Hits Netflix, Black Vietnam Veterans Recall the Real Injustices They Faced." *Time*, June 12, 2020. https://time .com/5852476/da-5-bloods-black-vietnam-veterans/.

"Court Confinements." *Baltimore Sun*, September 21, 1969.

"Curtain Lowering on Curley's Remarkable, Riotous Show." *Baltimore Sun*, September 16, 1990.

Fendrich, James M. "The Returning Black Vietnam-Era Veteran." *Social Service Review* 46 (1972): 60–75.

Geiselman A. W. "Slipshod Justice for Mental Cases." *Baltimore Sun*, September 28, 1969.

Herridge, Catherine. "Black Vietnam Veteran's Nearly 60-Year Wait for Medal of Honor Is Over." CBS News, February 14, 2023. https://www.cbsnews .com/news/black-vietnam-veterans-nearly-60-year-wait-for-medal-of-honor-is -over/.

Interim Report: The Present Status of the Criminal Insane of Maryland, 1952. S215, box 34, Department of Mental Hygiene Board of Review (General File) 1951–1961. Maryland State Archives.

Metzl, Jonathan. *The Protest Psychosis: How Schizophrenia Became a Black Disease*. Boston: Beacon, 2010.

Ornstein, Charles. "The Agent Orange Widows Club." ProPublica, December 28, 2016. https://www.propublica.org/article/the-agent-orange-widows-club.

Ornstein, Charles, Hannah Fresques, and Mike Hixenbaugh. "The Children of Agent Orange." ProPublica, December 16, 2016. https://www.propublica.org/article /the-children-of-agent-orange.

Report on the Mental Hospitals of the State of Maryland, 1949, Reports, T2811-1. Crownsville Hospital Center, Department of Health and Mental Hygiene (General File). Maryland State Archives.

Smith, Stuart S. "Plan to Put Prison Camp at Crownsville Questioned." *Baltimore Sun*, June 21, 1961.

Wolins, Martin, and Yochanan Wozner. "Deinstitutionalization and the Benevolent Asylum." *Social Service Review* 51, no. 4 (1977): 604-625.

Part Five
Chapter Seventeen: In the Balance

Author interview with Doug Struck. Virtual, October 29, 2021.

Author interview with Rodney Barnes. Los Angeles, December 16, 2021.

Author interview with Thomas and Barbara Arthur. Virtual, April 20, 2022.

Ax, Robert, and Thomas Fagan. *Corrections, Mental Health, and Social Policy: International Perspectives*. Springfield, IL: Charles C. Thomas, 2007.

Engel, Jonathan. "Deinstitutionalization in Maryland: A State's Response to Federal Legislation, 1945–1975." PhD dissertation, Yale University, 1994.

Gottschalk, Marie. "Cell Blocks & Red Ink: Mass Incarceration, the Great Recession and Penal Reform." *Daedalus* 139 (Summer 2010): 62–73.

Harcourt, Bernard E. "An Institutionalization Effect: The Impact of Mental Hospitalization and Imprisonment on Homicide in the United States, 1934–2001." *Journal of
   Legal Studies* 40 (January 2011): 39–83.

Harcourt, Bernard E. "From the Asylum to the Prison: Rethinking the Incarceration
   Revolution." *Texas Law Review* 84 (2006): 1751–1786.

Harcourt, Bernard E. "Reducing Mass Incarceration: Lessons from the Deinstitutionalization of Mental Hospitals in the 1960s." *Ohio State Journal of Criminal Law* 9
   (2011): 53–85.

LaGuerre, Diane Phillips, Lisa Phillips, Gregory McKenzie Phillips, Orlando
   McKenzie Phillips, and Muhammed Lloyd McKenzie Phillips. Letter to Antonia
   Hylton. "Life of George McKenzie Phillips," July 7, 2023.

"Mentally Ill Persons in Corrections." National Institute of Corrections, United
   States Department of Justice. [n.d.] Accessed February 20, 2015. http://nicic.gov
   /mentalillness.

Parsons, Anne E. "From Asylum to Prison: The Story of Lincoln, Illinois." *Journal of
   Illinois History* 15 (Winter 2011): 242–260.

Region III, Philadelphia Department of Health, Education, and Welfare and other Federal Agencies. "Deinstitutionalization of the Mentally Disabled in Maryland." United
   States General Accounting Office, Washington Regional Office, July 7, 1976. http://
   www.gao.gov/assets/200/191192.pdf.

Roth, Alisa. "The Truth About Deinstitutionalization." *The Atlantic*, May 25, 2021. https://
   www.theatlantic.com/health/archive/2021/05/truth-about-deinstitutionalization
   /618986/.

Struck, Doug. "6-Day Diary of Nothing: Time Meaningless in Hospital Ward." *Evening Capital*, October 8, 1975.

Struck, Doug. "Apathy of Hospital Staff Takes Its Toll on Patients." *Evening Capital*,
   October 9, 1975.

Struck, Doug. "Crownsville: Jail, Not Hospital." *Evening Capital*, October 6, 1975.

Struck, Doug. "Crownsville Changing in Keeping with Trend." *Evening Capital*, October 10, 1975.

Struck, Doug. "Crownsville's Boss: Do Outside Jobs Hinder His Effectiveness?" *Evening Capital*, October 17, 1975.

Struck, Doug. "Crownsville's History." *Evening Capital*, October 11, 1975.

Struck, Doug. "'Snake Pit' Image Lingers." *Evening Capital*, October 15, 1975.

Struck, Doug. "Underfunding Limits Staff: Experts Score Treatment." *Evening Capital*,
   October 13, 1975.

Struck, Doug. "What Is It Like Inside Crownsville?" *Evening Capital*, October 3, 1975.

Thompson, Heather Ann. "Why Mass Incarceration Matters: Rethinking Crisis,
   Decline, and Transformation in Postwar American History." *Journal of American History* 97 (December 2010): 703–734.

Ulle, Margaret B. Rep. *Humane Practices Commission.* Paul Lurz personal collection, n.d.

Ziedenberg, Jason, and Eric Lotke. *Tipping Point: Maryland's Overuse of Incarceration
   and the Impact on Public Safety.* Washington, D.C.: Justice Policy Institute, 2005.

Chapter Eighteen: Irredeemable or Incurable

"4 Crownsville Inmates Flee from Hospital: Escape Criminally Insane Ward; Doctor Calls Them 'Dangerous.'" *Baltimore Sun*, September 18, 1951.

Apperson, Jay. "Curtain Lowering on Curley's Remarkable, Riotous Show." *Baltimore Sun*, September 16, 1990.

Author interview with Paul Lurz. Annapolis, February 4, 2015.

Author interviews with Dr. Brian Sims. Virtual, January 16 and January 19, 2023.

"Baltimore City Public Schools History: From the Old Order to the New Order— Reasons and Results, 1957–1997." Baltimore City Public School System, https://web .archive.org/web/20040102085255/http://www.baltimorecityschools.org/About /History/From_the_oldorder1.asp.

"Bill to Commit Deranged Filed." *Baltimore Sun*, January 29, 1969.

"Court Confinements." *Baltimore Sun*, September 21, 1969.

"Crowding of Youths at Crownsville Told." *Baltimore Afro-American*, February 7, 1953.

Geiselman, A. W. "Slipshod Justice for Mental Cases." *Baltimore Sun*, September 28, 1969.

Harcourt, Bernard E. "An Institutionalization Effect: The Impact of Mental Hospitalization and Imprisonment on Homicide in the United States." *Journal of Legal Studies* 40 (January 2011): 39–83.

Harcourt, Bernard E. "Reducing Mass Incarceration: Lessons from the Deinstitutionalization of Mental Hospitals in the 1960s." *Ohio State Journal of Criminal Law* 9 (2011): 53–85.

Hirsch, Arthur. "Delegate, Physician Aris T. Allen Commits Suicide at 80." *Baltimore Sun*, September 29, 2021.

Interim Report: The Present Status of the Criminal Insane of Maryland, 1952. S215, box 34, Department of Mental Hygiene Board of Review (General File) 1951–1961. Maryland State Archives.

Lurz, Paul. Email message to author, February 21, 2015.

Metzl, Jonathan. *The Protest Psychosis: How Schizophrenia Became a Black Disease*. Boston: Beacon, 2010.

Parsons, Anne E. "From Asylum to Prison: The Story of Lincoln, Illinois." *Journal of Illinois History* 15 (Winter 2011): 242–260.

"Plan to Put Prison Camp at Crownsville Questioned." *Baltimore Sun*, June 21, 1961.

Report on the Mental Hospitals of the State of Maryland, 1949, Reports, T2811-1. Crownsville Hospital Center, Department of Health and Mental Hygiene (General File). Maryland State Archives.

Thompson, Heather Ann. "Why Mass Incarceration Matters: Rethinking Crisis, Decline, and Transformation in Postwar American History." *Journal of American History* 97 (December 2010): 703–734.

Wacquant, Loïc. "Class, Race & Hyperincarceration in Revanchist America." *Daedalus* 139 (Summer 2010): 74–90.

Weill Cornell Medical College. "The Rise and Decline of Psychiatric Hydrotherapy." Oskar Diethelm Library. http://www.cornellpsychiatry.org/history/osk_die_lib /hydrotherapy/default.htm.

Ziedenberg, Jason, and Eric Lotke. *Tipping Point: Maryland's Overuse of Incarceration and the Impact on Public Safety*. Washington, D.C.: Justice Policy Institute, 2005.

Chapter Nineteen: The Fire

Author interview with Gertrude and Faye Belt. Virtual, May 15, 2023.

Author interviews with Rev. Sonia King. Odenton, November 18, 2022, and May 12, 2023.

Chapter Twenty: Closing Crownsville

Author interview with Faye Belt. Annapolis, May 1, 2022.

Author interview with Joyce and Errol Phillip. Virtual, April 20, 2022.

Author interview with Steuart Pittman. Virtual, May 9, 2023.

Author interviews with Dr. Brian Sims. Virtual, January 13 and 19, 2023.

Author interviews with Janice Hayes-Williams. Anne Arundel County, April 29 and 30, 2022.

"Maryland Historical Trust NR-Eligibility Review Form." November 2, 2000.

Private performance memo with data from 2003 and 2004. Maryland Department of Health and Mental Hygiene, Services and Institutional Operations.

"Say My Name." Ceremony held in grounds of Crownsville Hospital, Crownsville, Maryland. April 30, 2022.

Epilogue: But for the Grace of God

Author interview with Dr. Brian Sims. Virtual, January 13, 2023.

Author interview with Dr. Tami Benton. Virtual, December 9, 2022.

Author interview with Faye Belt. Phone, May 15, 2023.

Author interview with Janice Hayes-Williams. Virtual, May 16, 2023.

Author interview with Pat Deegan. Virtual, January 16, 2023.

Cramer, Maria, and Chelsia Rose Marcius. "Man Dies on Subway After Another Rider Places Him in Chokehold." *New York Times*, May 2, 2023. https://www.nytimes.com/2023/05/02/nyregion/subway-chokehold-death.html.

McCarthy, Craig, Larry Celona, and Jorge Fitz-Gibbon. "Shocking Video Shows NYC Subway Passenger Putting Unhinged Man in Deadly Chokehold." *New York Post*, May 2, 2023. https://nypost.com/2023/05/02/shocking-video-shows-vagrant-being-choked-to-death-on-nyc-subway/.

Schiele, Jerome H., ed. *Social Welfare Policy: Regulation and Resistance Among People of Color*. Thousand Oaks, CA: SAGE Publications, Inc., 2011. Online at Sage Knowledge. https://doi.org/10.4135/9781452275185.

Swartz, Marvin S., Jeffrey W. Swanson, Henry J. Steadman, Pamela Clark Robbins, and John Monahan. *New York State Assisted Outpatient Treatment Program Evaluation*. Durham, NC: Duke University School of Medicine, 2009.

INDEX

NOTE: *Italic page numbers* indicate photographs